HYPNOBIRTHING COURSE

Essential Guide To A Pain-Free, Calm & Safe Childbirth Using Hypnosis + Mindfulness Techniques, Filled With The Best Meditation, Breathing, And Visualization Secrets

TABLE OF CONTENTS

CHAPTER TWELVE ---130

CHAPTER THIRTEEN: WELCOME HOME -----------------------136

CONCLUSION --140

INTRODUCTION

You've probably picked up this book because you're pregnant – or your partner is – and you've heard the word "hypnobirthing" tossed around a lot but aren't sure what it entails or if it's something you should spend your hard-earned time or money on.

So, first and foremost, let me reassure you that hypnobirthing does not include being hypnotized and has nothing to do with hippies – or even hippos! In reality, hypnobirthing is nothing out of the ordinary, except for the name, which is ironic. Most contemporary hypnobirthing teachers would accept that the practice of hypnobirthing could use a rebranding. There's no denying that the term "Hypno" scares people away and causes them to have doubts about what hypnobirthing is all about.

Hypnobirthing, in my opinion, is better represented as the psychology of childbirth. It's a lot like sports psychology, in reality. Women must prepare psychologically for labour and imminent motherhood in order to get the most out of the experience, just as athletes must prepare mentally as well as physically to improve their results.

Essentially, hypnobirthing is a form of antenatal education, an evidence-based and logical approach to childbirth. It - surprise you to learn that it is actually more scientific than anything else! This book will teach you about the physiology of birth, which refers to how the body functions on a muscular and hormonal level during labour. This should increase your self-assurance and make it easier to trust that your body knows what it's doing. Importantly, you will learn how to work with your body (rather than against it) to ensure that the proper hormones are made, making labour more productive and comfortable for both you and your infant.

You'll learn that remaining calm and relaxed is crucial and that this has a direct and positive effect on the outcome of your birth. You'll learn how to use the hypnobirthing toolkit, which includes breathing techniques, visualizations, guided calming exercises, light-touch massage, positive affirmations, and other techniques, to quickly and easily access a state of deep relaxation. You'll also learn how to make educated decisions using a straightforward structure, so you can confidently manage your birth – and any twists and turns it can bring – with the help of practical aids that keep you calm and in charge.

Importantly, hypnobirthing is not appropriate for every type of birth, just as it is not appropriate for every type of woman. Hypnobirthing is suitable for any woman who has a baby in her uterus (you do not need to follow any specific school of thought) and for any form of birth (from a natural water birth without intervention or pain relief through to an unplanned cesarean). Many women come to hypnobirthing hoping for a vaginal birth, but I always tell them that the logistics of how a baby enters the world are unimportant in the long run compared to how the mother felt during the experience because feelings last a lifetime. This is why a positive birth experience is so critical, as it benefits mothers, infants, and entire families for the rest of their lives. A happy birth is well known for lowering a woman's risk of postnatal depression (PND) and posttraumatic stress disorder (PTSD) (PTSD). Giving birth and being a mother to a small child is a life-changing event for a woman, whether it's her first or fourth child, which is why birth is so important. Even if motherhood is all about winging it, investing some time in planning for a healthy birth is still worthwhile. In this book, you'll learn about inductions and caesareans, as well as how to use hypnobirthing methods to make every birth positive.

So, what exactly qualifies as a happy birth? A positive birth, in my opinion, is one in which a woman feels empowered rather than traumatized, one in which the mother's desires are respected, she is listened to, and she is calm, optimistic, and aware during the process. There isn't just one form of birth: water birth, home birth, induction, and cesarean. Every birth has the potential to be a positive experience.

The aim of the hypnobirthing program is to assist women – and their birth partners – in having positive birth experiences. Learning about hypnobirthing is useful for birth partners as well because it provides them with realistic resources to aid Mum's relaxation, a structure to help them ask the right questions, information about how to create a birth-friendly atmosphere, and a detailed to-do list, so they know how to assist Mum during childbirth better. Instead of feeling anxious and like a spare part in the room, hypnobirthing makes birth partners feel calm, motivated and prepared for the job. Giving birth is a team effort in hypnobirthing, not a solo endeavour, so make sure you share this book with your birth partner.

Finally, hypnobirthing helps your baby by ensuring a gentle entrance into the world and a mother who is calm, optimistic, and happy. A healthy birth provides the best possible start for everyone.

From beginning to end, this book will cover everything you'd learn on a hypnobirthing course. As you advance through the book and learn more, you'll feel as if you're finishing a course – albeit a fun one!

CHAPTER ONE

WHAT IS MINDFUL HYPNOBIRTHING?

Thousands of women around the world have used mindful hypnobirthing, a rare mixture of hypnosis and mindfulness, to have a positive birth experience. Deeply embedding optimistic, calm, and encouraging thoughts about your baby's birth will help your body react well during labour.

Mothers who have used this approach still remark about how peacefully excited they were about their baby's birth, rather than apprehensive or nervous.

Both hypnosis and mindfulness will assist you in connecting with the part of yourself that is not conscious. This is special to mindful hypnobirthing and allows you to change your mindset from one of fear, anxiety, or apprehension to one of calm, optimistic anticipation. Mindful hypnobirthing differs from basic relaxation methods in that it works on a deeper level than relaxation to adjust your reactions to birth, which is essentially far more effective.

Using hypnosis to prepare for birth will benefit you not only during labour and delivery but also in other aspects of your life for several years.

MINDFULNESS AND HYPNOSIS

What is hypnosis, and how does it work?

Hypnosis is a normal state of consciousness. It happens at least twice a day: when you go to sleep and when you wake up in the morning.

It's the cozy spot you go to when you're half-awake and half-asleep when you're on the verge of falling asleep. It's been compared to daydreaming by some. This brain condition is also known as alpha (light hypnosis) or theta (deep hypnosis). It's amazing as a therapy. Hypnosis can quickly transport an individual into a healthy state of mind, allowing them to overcome phobias, habits, and behaviours that have kept them from living a happy life.

When you use hypnosis, you gain access to areas of your mind that are normally hidden from view. All of your life experiences, everything you've been told, done, and learned is stored in your brain, but it's always accessed automatically and without your knowledge. In fact, you can only concentrate on a few small pieces of information at a time.

Hypnosis is a treatment with a specific purpose in mind. When I use hypnosis, I always ask my clients how they want to be, and then we use very specific methods to get there.

The way a hypnotherapist initiates change is heavily influenced by language; it is often motivating and very precise in its pattern and structure. You are using specific words to make reading Mindful Hypnobirthing a hypnotic experience in and of itself! You may not know it, but when you read a book, you enter a trance state in which you use your imagination in a variety of ways. Because of the way this book is published, you can make profound and unconsciously meaningful changes simply by reading or listening to it.

What is the concept of mindfulness?

Mindfulness is a unique experience. Rather than concentrating on a distant target, you've chosen to concentrate on the here and now. Mindfulness is a technique for approaching life with mindfulness, transparency, and loving-kindness. You can develop a sense of insight, inner peace, and gentle compassion by being conscious of how you perceive your life. Being conscious entails being aware of one's surroundings and present moment experience. It's not as easy as recognizing that you're sleeping, doing the dishes, or showering. When you eat, you may find yourself worrying about things, conversing with your wife, or watching television. You are aware that you are feeding, but your focus is not on the act of eating. If you eat mindfully, you'd be conscious of the knife's edge as it cuts the potato, the feeling of the potato hitting your lips, chewing the potato while paying attention to the taste, and then swallowing.

When you're doing something routine, your mind can wander; mindfulness is about bringing your focus back to what you're doing. You are not dwelling in the past or projecting into the future while you are mindful. You are in the moment, enjoying being alive and alert to your senses.

What's the Difference Between Hypnosis and Mindfulness?

When you practice mindfulness meditation or hypnosis, you will reach an alpha or theta brain state, which is a naturally occurring altered state of mind that is more concentrated. If you use hypnosis or practice mindfulness, you are quieting the chattering portion of your mind that loses clarity and concentration at times.

Hypnosis is a technique for inducing a theta brain state, in which you can access thoughts and emotions that are normally unnoticed, in order to alter a negative or problematic pattern of action by projecting into the future or reframing reactions to past events. Using breath awareness or self-hypnosis, a person may enter a trance-like, or hypnotic, state on their own.

The main distinction between the two methods is how you stay in that state. Mindfulness meditation will help you focus on what is happening right now. Instead, when you're in hypnosis, you're focused on a target, either in the future or on a previous experience, in order to change your reaction to it. The goal of hypnosis is to alter an unpleasant or obstructive behaviour pattern, while the goal of mindfulness is to accept a feeling or behaviour. The results of mindfulness and hypnosis may often be very similar.

11

Many who use these strategies on a daily basis report less anxiety, depression, and tension, as well as a better ability to handle stress.

In certain areas of medicine, evidence of the effects of hypnotherapy and mindfulness is now so clear that their use is recommended to treat insomnia, irritable bowel syndrome (IBS), anxiety, and depression. Both approaches are increasingly being recognized in conventional psychological treatment models for the advantages they have in our daily lives.

HYPNOSIS FOR PREGNANCY

Is Hypnobirthing a New Concept?

You might be shocked to learn that hypnosis for childbirth is not a new concept. In 1858, James Braid dubbed the "Father of Hypnotherapy," published a paper on using hypnotherapy to induce a woman to give birth early for medical reasons. In the 1950s, the Soviet Union compiled the results of large and effective hypnosis for the birth program, which revealed that hypnotherapy reduced pain in 83 percent of births.

In the 1950s, Magonet, a doctor and hypnotherapist, predicted that "hypnotherapy in antenatal clinics would be regarded as just as critical as pelvic scales, blood pressure readings, and urine examinations." Despite the fact that Magonet's vision was not realized, hypnotherapy is becoming more widely used in pregnancy planning. It is now more often referred to as hypnobirthing. Much different hypnosis for birth approaches have developed over the years, each slightly different in content, delivery, duration, and design but all based on the same philosophy: If the mother is fearless and trusts her body to do what it does naturally, she will have the best birth possible.

Early approaches to hypnosis for birth were focused on pain control, but now the underlying idea is that birth is not something to be dreaded but rather something to embrace and enjoy fully. After all, you can only be able to count on one hand how many times you do it! Hypnobirthing will boost your morale and make you realize – both consciously and subconsciously – that you are capable of giving birth to your baby and having a positive experience. This means that when you go into labour, you'll have controlled excitement and a relaxed body as a natural reaction.

Hypnosis for Childbirth: Different Approaches

There are two methods of hypnosis for childbirth. This book will provide you with the strategies to help whatever method you choose. The first method is more conventional, relying on hypnosis as a pain-relieving technique. If they haven't had advanced training in the relationship between the body and the mind after birth, most hypnotherapists will use this method. Many women find these approaches to be extremely beneficial, and they have proven to be effective in treating chronic pain. These techniques are also used in Hypno-anesthesiology, which is a type of anesthesia used for operations, minor surgical procedures, and dental surgery.

The second method, which is now more widely used for birth, is even more systematic and considers the physiology and psychology of birth as a whole. You'll discover how unconsciously held thoughts can cause anxiety and pain in your body. This method focuses on addressing any fears you might have about giving birth and allowing your body to do what it was created to do. When this method works, the body produces endorphins, which are natural painkillers, and you do not need to use pharmacological pain relief. Even more significantly, in my experience, this strategy is hugely inspiring, fostering resilience and a positive experience—the ideal base for those early parenting days.

THOUGHTS, BOTH CONSCIOUS AND UNCONSCIOUS

Hypnosis and other types of mind therapy operate on a far deeper level than our everyday consciousness. Your brain can be processing thousands of different items in rapid succession at any given time and is always on the move. It is, however, difficult to be conscious of all of the information your brain is processing at any given time.

Without you consciously noticing it, your subconscious is continuously processing and filtering messages from the world around you. Perception without knowledge is what it's called.

When Derren Brown, a well-known mentalist and illusionist, builds up a belief or implants a suggestion into someone's mind before performing a "mind-reading trick," he uses this psychological mechanism to his advantage. Intentionally or unconsciously, we shape opinions, emotions, and feelings based on what we have absorbed during our lives.

Your conscious awareness can access reference systems and retrieve information as needed, but it can only handle a small amount at a time. This means that many of your answers are automatic and can occur without your knowledge. Frequently, the body reacts without you even realizing what you're doing. Consider how we ride a bike, make a cup of tea, or brush our teeth. These are all automatically learned answers that we don't have to worry about when we do them.

Later in the book, you'll discover why these brain-body interactions have such an effect on how you give birth. You'll also learn how to modify and adjust certain reference structures for the better so that your automated physical responses aid in the rapid progress of your labour while keeping you relaxed and focused.

HOW DOES HYPNOSIS MAKE YOU FEEL?

When you're in hypnosis, rest assured that you'll still be in command. I can't make you eat onion or cluck like a chicken. Stage hypnosis has done hypnotherapy a disservice; it's always a sly manipulation of magic, illusion, psychology, and hypnosis, and it's nothing like the hypnotherapy practiced by thousands of skilled hypnotherapists throughout the nation. In reality, it's been said that all hypnosis is self-hypnosis, which means you're still in control.

You will benefit from hypnosis even though you're not in a trance. This is referred to as "non-state hypnosis." Some well-known hypnotherapists employ a strong method of conversation hypnosis, using distinct patterns of language to facilitate progress.

You can feel as though you are resting or dreaming if you use state hypnosis. You will have the option to open your eyes at any time. Non-state hypnosis and state hypnosis are also experienced during hypnobirthing.

This is the best form of hypnosis to practice for birth because your delivery would be much faster if your muscles are relaxed, calm, and working together. When listening to the tracks included in the novel, you'll notice the same thing.

The majority of people are taken aback by how calming hypnosis is and how well their bodies react to it. You can feel as though you are fully conscious of your surroundings or as if you have fallen asleep; any feeling is ideal. You might feel heavier, as if your body were sinking, or as if you're drifting. Trust that your mind will guide you into hypnosis in a way that is relaxing and appropriate for you; the more you practice and trust the method, the more profoundly relaxed you will become.

Continue even if it doesn't seem to be working for you; simply encourage yourself to let go. Perhaps you should seek out a location where you can feel less self-conscious and more confident. It will all come together at once, and you will be shocked at how easy it is to let go and enjoy the deep state of hypnotic relaxation.

BIRTHING WITH MINDFULNESS

Birth should be approached with awareness. It's an opportunity to set aside preconceived notions and desires and focus on the present moment with your body and your kid.

Being conscious during your birth means being linked to your body's experience and rhythm in each moment. When you are in the moment, you are able to step away from any worries you might have had in the past and back to fears you may have had in the future. You allow yourself to yield to your deep confidence in yourself and your innate ability to tap into your own inner resources and strength in the present moment.

You will be able to be more in contact with what you need at the moment if you are mindful of and moment and present. You'll be able to be at ease with discomfort, curious about the power of your experience, and interested in it. Many women who have learned hypnotherapy for birth find that mindfulness is all they need and that sitting with their breath and being concentrated on it is all they require. It's in this state of mindful consciousness that you'll be able to respond to your birthing body's needs. You become dependent on your breathing while you sit with your breath. Now try this:

Concentrate on your breathing while closing your eyes. When you breathe in, note how cool the air feels and how it expands your chest. And, when you breathe out, note the warmth of the air as your chest falls. Breathing in, coolness rises in your chest; breathing out, warmth falls in your chest. Continue doing so for a few minutes, concentrating on the sensations of inhaling and exhaling. If your mind wanders, simply return to your breath by repeating the mantra "breathing in and breathing out."

Any feelings you get during labour and delivery are signals from your body. Allowing the body to let go and open up by turning towards those stimuli and accepting them at the moment as something constructive – enjoying them rather than fighting them. This knowledge will motivate you to change positions or move in a specific manner. Being in the moment strengthens the bond between your body and mind, allowing you to have a better sense of how to roll, rock, and sway during labour.

THE IDEAL COMBINATION FOR A HAPPY BIRTH

For a healthy birth experience, hypnosis and mindfulness are excellent combinations. Your hypnosis training will aid in the processing of latent fears, helping your body to relax and react to labour in a natural way during the day. During labour, mindfulness will help you stay connected and in contact with what you, your body, and your baby needs. Hypnosis and mindfulness should be combined with other lessons you've taken, such as active birth or pregnancy yoga.

ASSISTING YOU IN MAINTAINING THE BIRTHING ZONE

You'll learn how to remain focused in your birthing zone with mindful hypnobirthing. Your birthing zone is a normal state of mind that occurs during labour and delivery. You spontaneously enter your birthing zone if you are fearless, calmly excited, and accepting of your body and birth.

Women may appear disorganized during birth, according to midwives. Many mothers who have given birth several times claim they were in a zone during childbirth and were unaware of what was going on around them. Since they were in their birthing zone, which is different from our usual levels of consciousness, women seldom remember the specifics of their baby's birth.

Your brain waves slow down during labour. Feeling exhausted, daydreaming, being in hypnosis, or using mindful meditation may be how you perceive this. Hypnosis and mindfulness both work well for birth because they help you remain in your birthing environment or return to it if anything disturbs or brings you out of it. They will assist you if you simply need anything to help you stay concentrated and focused. In the following pages, you'll hear a lot more about your birthing zone.

PREGNANCY BENEFITS

If you use hypnotherapy to prepare for your birth and practice every day, you will notice positive side effects such as being calmer, sleeping better, and feeling more mentally at ease. Women say that once they start listening to their hypnosis tracks or meditating, their insomnia and heartburn vanish.

Hypnotherapy and meditation, unlike many other pregnancy therapies, are non-invasive and can be used safely to help relieve symptoms like heartburn, nausea, and insomnia. They can also be used to de-stress, relax, and let go, giving you time to interact with and focus on your child.

You are profoundly relaxed when you are in a hypnotic or aware state. When you use hypnotherapy, the conscious mind drifts away, and any bothersome or troubling thoughts fade away as you relax and allow yourself to be directed by someone else's soothing voice. Being conscious will help you become more aware of the present moment, your body, and your growing baby. It can be a very satisfying way to bond with your baby, as well as the physical changes that are taking place in your body. The more you become used to living in such states and feeling secure in your environment while pregnant, the easier it will be to extend them to birth.

Your muscles relax, and your baby always moves in reaction to these positive feelings as you enter this deep hypnosis state. How much does your baby begin to move just when you're falling asleep? Since your muscles relax as you mentally let go, your baby has more room to shift and stretch. The time you spend using mind stimulation methods will help both you and your kid.

You can teach yourself to go through self-hypnosis and use clear visualizations to help handle something that is disturbing or upsetting you by using the strategies in this book. Listening to hypnosis tracks is a quick and easy way to reap the benefits of these therapies while pregnant.

WHAT WOULD MY MIDWIFE'S REACTION BE?

When you discussed hypnobirthing with your midwife a few years ago, you may have gotten a raised eyebrow. More and more midwives are seeing the benefits firsthand and accepting those births, thanks to the thousands of people who are practicing and experiencing births using this method. Many people are now teaching it to others.

You should have a group midwife in your planning if you have one. Discuss how you'd like her to assist you and ask her medical questions to help you better understand your birth options. If you're getting your baby in the hospital, make sure your birth preferences match your use of hypnosis and ask staff to assist you in creating the right atmosphere.

Hypnosis training will help you create a positive relationship between your body and mind during labour by working with your unconscious. Mindfulness will assist you in tuning in to your instinctive body and recognizing cues to move your body in a way that will assist your baby is getting into the ideal place for birth. At a deep unconscious level, mindful hypnobirthing will shift your negative perceptions about your body and birth, helping you to feel focused and in control.

CHAPTER TWO

THE BENEFITS OF A MINDFUL HYPNOBIRTH

Preparing for a conscious hypnobirthing has advantages for you, your wife, and your child. Unlike several other antenatal preparations, this one is special. It's not all about unwinding. You may be shocked to learn that the elements of emotional and mental readiness call attention to facets of the birth or parenting that you weren't even aware of before. It will prepare you in more ways than you can imagine, and you will be far more in control when you are emotionally focused and powerful.

MUM'S ADVANTAGES

Motherhood and Childbirth

Whether giving birth excites or frightens you, the closer you get to it, the more you'll concentrate on it rather than your pregnancy or the first few weeks after your baby is born. Your body expands and grows during the months you are pregnant.

You may be looking forward to seeing your baby's movements and feeling your bump. Week by week, you could be tracking your baby's development in books or on the internet, seeing how he or she changes and grows. How much time have you spent contemplating your body's changes during pregnancy? What percentage of your attention should you devote to such drastic changes?

Consider how your body expands to accommodate your infant, developing an internal life support system that includes a heart and lungs, as well as tiny feet, eyes, and a brain. It's amazing, and it does it without you even realizing it. As your body softens and grows, you can notice stretching, tweaks, and pain, but embrace these as part of your pregnancy journey.

Pregnancy-related anxiety does occur, but not to the same extent as birth-related anxiety. According to some surveys, four out of every five women are concerned about giving birth. This means that there's an 80% chance you're worried or anxious about giving birth. What is the reason for this? To begin with, many modern women are unaware of the physiology of birth; they are not taught about their bodies or the amazing physical changes that enable our babies to be born.

During your pregnancy, you will have a strong feeling that your life is about to change and that you have no influence over how such changes will occur. On an unconscious level, this can be rather disturbing, even though you don't feel the need to examine or think about it consciously.

Clinicians often overlook the 'thoughts and feelings' aspect of birth. They can separate the physical and psychological aspects of birth, viewing it solely as a medical event. However, the physical essence of birth is intertwined with your mental well-being before and after your birth.

ACCEPTING BIRTH AS A STAGE OF LIFE

Birthmarks, a turning point process that began when your baby was born and will continue beyond birth, into childhood, adolescence, and adulthood. It's a turning point and a transitional period in your relationship with your son. Your baby will no longer be safe inside you, and the special bond you have with him or her when he or she is still in your womb will change. After your baby is born, your bond will always be there, but it will shift and develop.

Unconsciously, women sense the impending transition. Giving birth is more than just bringing your child into the world; it is also a means of release and separation, the first of many that will occur in your child's life. It will happen again at nursery or pre-school, and in a different way when they enter primary school, and again when they enter secondary school, and eventually when they leave home. Understanding this and preparing to make the necessary changes is an essential part of birth planning. Acceptance of the transition into motherhood comes from a willingness to let go and yield to the experience of birth.

Birth is a time of personal development and transformation. Giving life is a life-changing experience that can change you from the inside out.

This may, understandably, trigger an implicit sense of sorrow or unease. This is particularly true in the final stages of pregnancy, just before the birth of the infant.

Birth will teach you about your own capabilities and power. What better way to prepare for motherhood than this? Young men are still undergoing initiation ceremonies into adulthood in many cultures around the world, which measure their mental and physical stamina and take them further into themselves than they have ever gone before. Many people consider birth to be the female counterpart to this life stage.

Take a moment to reflect on your life and the events that have shaped you into the person you are today. Those moments are frequently ones that have tested you; they might have been thrust upon you or ones that you choose. They are, most importantly, moments that have propelled you forward, making you stronger and more conscious of your own skills. This is what birth is: a once-in-a-lifetime experience that you would be able to reflect on and think, "Wow, I did that." What an amazing experience and accomplishment.'

You can hit a point during childbirth where you believe you can't do anymore. There will be times when you doubt yourself and need to seek assistance. Others may wish to assist you, possibly with narcotics, which may cause you to become distracted or disrupt your rhythm. Drugs can also dull the birthing experience by preventing you from responding to how your body needs to shift or react during labour in order to help your baby get into the best place for birth. But it's at this stage if you're well supported, that you'll be able to go beyond what you think you're capable of. Now is the time when you'll find out what you're really capable of doing.

YOUR PARTNER'S ADVANTAGES

Getting in Touch with Your Feelings and Emotions

It's possible that your partner has trained for their realistic function at birth. For example, they will be prepared to load your birth bag into the car, know where the hospital's parking is, ensure you have food and water during labour, and possibly know how to massage you during the birth.

However, they, like you, will begin emotionally planning in the months leading up to the birth. They can understand the importance of caring for a family, as well as being a parent and role model. They may be ecstatic, but they may also be concerned about how they will care for you during the birth.

Your partner may feel more emotionally involved with your pregnancy and the birth of your baby if you have a conscientious hypnobirthing. Taking the time to plan together, expressing your thoughts and concerns in a thoughtful and reflective manner will make a big difference in how you prepare for parenthood.

Understanding the distinctions between functional and emotional readiness may be beneficial to a spouse. If your partner understands the importance of giving you space and letting go of their concerns about the birth, it will be a huge help to you. By resolving these concerns during pregnancy, you will be able to develop a stronger bond at birth that is based on love rather than fear.

Birth can also put a spouse to the test, and it's an excellent opportunity to practice mindfulness and let go of preconceived notions.

BABY'S ADVANTAGES

In the womb, a Soothing Life

Your baby will go through a transformation because they are so warm and relaxed in their watery world with the muffled sound of your heartbeat to soothe them. How would you feel if you landed on an alien planet with just a few resemblances of your own?

Practicing conscientious hypnobirthing during pregnancy also helps to prepare the baby for birth. Your baby picks up on your feelings and atmosphere, so if you're relaxed, so is your baby. Your baby will leap in response to a loud bang. When you go to bed at night and snuggle into your bed, your baby begins to move in response to you, releasing the stress of the day.

Perinatal psychology, or the study of the infant's brain and maternal brain before and after birth, is becoming increasingly popular as a field of study. For those of us who have experienced stress or depression during or after pregnancy, this study may be troubling at times. It's important for women to understand, however, that when you take time to relax and let go, your baby benefits greatly. If you work a demanding job, consider the benefits of taking breaks for your baby during the day. Even five minutes of listening to your pregnancy affirmations (the second hypnosis track for this) can have a significant impact.

From the womb to the world

The planning you've done will aid your baby's response when you go into labour. Consider your baby in your womb, where they've been for nine months, listening to your heartbeat and the muffled noises outside, their eyes closed but mindful of bright light shining on your abdomen. Your waters have protected the baby from knocks and bumps. Even before labour begins, each contraction, tightening, or pressure feels like a firm massage, palpating and awakening the nerve endings in your baby's arms and legs slowly and gently. You will feel calm and happy in a caring and compassionate atmosphere during a hypnobirthing. Your baby will pick up on this and will benefit from your normal endorphins. With each contraction, your baby travels down through your vaginal canal and is finally born into a world that is very different from the one they are used to. Bright lights and loud noises, rather than the darkness and muffled sounds they are used to, are very common, even in undisturbed birth. A baby may be removed from their mother, rubbed down with a towel, and placed on a collection of cold, hard scales. In that split second, all sense of familiarity vanishes. In that new and strange location, only your voice, your partner's voice, and your scent are familiar anchors.

Assuring that your baby's entry into the world is as gentle and peaceful as possible will help to settle and calm them. As a mother, you can help to reduce interference as much as possible by being conscious, but also by trusting our bodies, taking responsibility for our births, and being aware of our options.

It's important to make your birth as stress-free as possible for both you and your infant. You will do so by concentrating on how your mental state affects your actions, experiences, and physical well-being during labour.

Even if your birth does not go as planned, your ability to remain calm and centred has a positive effect on your infant. The oxygen supply to your baby is decreased when you are anxious for a long time during labour. Your baby's heart will beat faster if you are nervous, according to research; if you are comfortable, centred, and calm, your baby will benefit.

CHAPTER THREE

GETTING READY FOR A MINDFUL HYPNOBIRTH

Hypnobirthing needs dedication. When you decide to use mindful hypnobirthing to prepare for your birth, you must do more than just read the book and practice the techniques once. You'll need to set aside time to learn how to use these techniques before your body has mastered them without your input. This is known as conditioning, and conditioning is a learned response; the more you do something, the more your body responds without the involvement of your mind.

Pavlov's dogs, a successful experiment, famously discovered how to get the birth brain into condition conditioning. Ivan Pavlov, a physiologist, was interested in learning more about learned and automatic behaviour. Pavlov rang a bell every time he gave food to his dogs in this experiment. Simply ringing the bell would cause the dogs to salivate for a short time. This allowed psychologists to see how a learned association could trigger a physical response in the body.

To show conditioning and connection, a well-known hypnotherapist used what he called the lemon sherbet experiment. This is something you can do right now. You can either read it first and then do the exercise, or you can make your partner, or a friend read it to you as you close your eyes. If you don't like lemon, replace it with something else you like. Let's use orange as an example.

Close your eyes and see yourself holding an orange sherbet. Keep an eye on the weight and pressure of the orange sherbet in your palm. Take a look at the orange sherbet and imagine how good it would taste. Imagine taking the orange sherbet in your other hand and putting it in your mouth. When you turn the orange sherbet in your mouth, be mindful of the sharpness of the orange taste. Change the orange sherbet from one side of your mouth to the other, then dissolve or crunch it while paying attention to the sensations and flavours in your mouth.

You will notice that your mouth is producing saliva. You may have even pursed your lips as you imagined the orange's sourness. Even if the orange sherbet in your mouth isn't really there, your body is reacting to the idea. Your training will teach your body to automatically react in a positive and comfortable manner to certain ideas, emotions, feelings, surroundings, and people during labour via conditioning.

PERFECTION COMES WITH PRACTICE.

You should make an effort to follow some of the methods taught in the book on a daily basis. Women who have gotten the most out of the therapies have been dedicated to listening to their hypnosis tracks and doing their exercises with and without their partners. You'll gain trust as you become more familiar with the strategies you'll learn in the book. You will not only be able to use them to help you remain calm and centred, but you will also have the confidence to adjust and modify them to fit your needs. The picture of the baby surfing is from a mother who attended my class; she had really internalized the techniques and had a surfing baby on the wall during her labour.

Hypnosis has the ability to harness your own ideas and emotions and use them to alter your feelings and reactions. I don't know what your personal feelings and opinions about birth are, but I do know that the methods in this book are described in such a way that you will be able to adapt and adjust them to suit the type of birth you are planning.

Daily practice will aid you in this endeavour. Other images, symbols, or methods can come to mind while you practice; if this happens, use them.

If possible, practice with your birth partner. It will help you become more accustomed to their voice and touch, and they will gain trust in their use of the techniques. If your partner is unavailable, ask a friend to assist you. Setting aside time with your partner at least once a week can be a wonderful way for you to prepare together and for your partner to become more conscious of your pregnancy and your baby.

HOW TO BUILD A PRACTICE AREA?

Find a quiet place where you won't be interrupted to practice the strategies in this book. Before going to bed, many women enjoy doing one of the mindfulness or hypnosis exercises. This is a perfect choice because you'll be less likely to be disturbed, and the hypnosis tracks will help you sleep better!

POSITIONS FOR PRACTICE

You will train in a variety of positions. While it is very relaxing to listen to music when lying down on your left side, you do not have to do so all of the time. You should practice the relaxation or hypnosis exercises in a variety of positions.

Both of these positions are helpful in getting your baby into a good place for labour and are very comfortable. All of the positions you specialize in are excellent for labour as well.

You can do some of the exercises in basic yoga positions that feel relaxed if you're just doing yoga as a means of training. This is a good option for light relaxation exercises and visualizations, as well as listening to hypnosis tracks. Since the birth planning track is 30 minutes long, keep in mind that you'll have to hold the spot for that long. Since the pregnancy or birth affirmations are much shorter, you might find it easier to listen to them when in a yoga pose.

Consider getting into the sitting positions as much as possible in your daily life, whether at work or at home. Don't overlook the value of maintaining good posture when pregnant. It is easier for your baby to get into place when you are in good positions. If your baby is in a good spot, labour would be much faster and smoother. When you relax, be particularly aware of your location because when your abdominal muscles relax, the baby tends to move more.

When you get used to learning, it may be beneficial to try it out in different environments and put yourself to the test in more noisy situations, such as at work, with other children, or even when waiting in line at the store. You'll notice that you're becoming more expert at turning your focus inwards and shutting off, as well as letting go of sounds and noises. You should listen to the exercises while riding the train to work, in a quiet space at work, or while your other children are sleeping. Some women prefer to practice in the bathtub or in the open air. It doesn't matter where you go as long as you feel safe, confident, and at ease. You can learn how to safely and rapidly float in and out of hypnosis by practicing at various times of the day and in noisier environments. Perfect labour planning.

SETTING YOUR BIRTH GOALS

Hypnosis is all about concentration and direction, so you must know where you're going, or you'll get sidetracked. Clients who want to experience those emotions should set a target for themselves and work toward it. Set your target and determine how you want to experience your birth to chart your path.

What are the most important things to you? You might want to be more in charge; you might want to be more confident; you might want to be calm; you might want to let go more easily. The strategies you use will help you remain concentrated and centred during labour by forming strong roots.

Assume you're a tree blowing in the wind. The wind will blow a gale or a gentle breeze, but your roots will remain strong, and you will be able to bend and sway because you were well prepared. The strategies are your roots, but they need to be nurtured, which you can do with careful planning. You can remain rooted and calm with a deep conviction that you are solid, focused, and secure instead of being blown around and afraid of being uprooted.

LISTENING TO THE HYPNOSIS RECORDINGS

Up until weeks 28–32, listen to the birth planning, pregnancy affirmations, and birth affirmations at least three times a week. You would want to listen to them every day for the rest of your life.

You will be in a deeper part of yourself after 28–32 weeks. Perhaps you're planning for the birth even if you're not aware of it. You might sense a change in your emotions that you can't put into words, or you might consciously begin to think about the birth ahead of you if you can turn to use all three tracks every day at this stage. It's fine to play them back-to-back for a 40-minute relaxing session. The hypnosis tracks are full of suggestions that aid in the formation of strong roots in your tree, as well as the development of your unconscious confidence and trust in the birthing process.

When driving or running equipment, do not listen to the hypnosis songs

You'll understand why after you've listened to them a few times. It's cool if you feel like you're falling asleep. It may seem that way during hypnosis, but it is simply your thought brain turning off. And if you do fall asleep, your mind will continue to process messages, so take advantage of the rest. No matter how profoundly people are hypnotized, they will still wake up and return to the room when they want to.

If possible, listen to the hypnosis tracks with stereo headphones since they use a hypnosis technique known as dual induction, which benefits greatly from stereo headphones.

It's important to remember that hypnosis is all about conditioning, repetition, and association. Mindfulness is about getting acquainted with the body's rhythms. Daily practice will allow your body to react while your mind remains calm, concentrated, and comfortable in your birthing zone. Decide how you want to give birth, and set aside a time and place to begin your mindful hypnobirthing journey.

CHAPTER FOUR

GETTING TO KNOW YOUR BIRTHING ZONE

Your brain waves slow down while you're in your birthing environment. It's a state that everybody is familiar with, and it's close to that state where you're not quite awake but not quite asleep. Since they were deep inside their birthing region, many mothers don't recall all of the specifics of their births. In your birthing zone, you lose track of time and focus on what's going on inside your body rather than what's going on outside. The human part of you avoids interfering by worrying about it and lets the animal part of you do it naturally, as it has for thousands of years for your forefathers.

This is a normal condition for many women during childbirth, and it could be the same for you. Other women can need strategies to help them remain in their comfort zone, particularly if they are thrown out of it. A noisy noise, an intrusion, or a change of scenery may all be examples. Hypnosis and mindfulness activities, as well as love and care, will help you stay in your birthing zone – or get back into it.

You are quieting down the part of your brain that is alert and chatty as you enter your birthing region. The inner narrator refers to the part of the brain that is always thinking and questioning why, how, and what. When you slow down this part of your brain, you depend on automatic responses from your old brain, which is the part of your brain that knows how to give birth, just like all other mammals.

THE NARRATOR INSIDE

The inner narrator, also known as the monkey mind or the chattering chimp, is a complex part of our brain that is different from that of other mammals. Our mind, according to the Buddha, is likened to a monkey: Much like a monkey grabbing a branch while swinging through the trees.

It grabs another branch after letting go of the first. It grabs another one after letting go of the first. It grabs another one after letting go of the first. Similarly, during the day and at night, what we call "mind," "intellect," or "consciousness" emerges as one thing and vanishes as another.

The neocortex, or new brain, is the part of our brain that acts in this manner. It's in control of a lot of things, but the elements of logic, self-awareness, conscious thinking and language have the most influence on how we perceive birth.

During labour, we need to minimize activity in our neocortex. It's the part we turn off when we sleep, meditate, or use hypnosis, which is why the strategies you'll learn are so effective. This is referred to as "bypassing the critical mind" in hypnosis. Your old brain is where your birthing zone is. The instinctive animal – the lioness inside – awakens when the neo-cortex becomes still and quiet. This is the section of the body that knows how to give birth.

HOW THINKING OBSTRUCTS A FANTASTIC BIRTH

Self-awareness is stored in our neocortex and can be troublesome during childbirth. The act of giving birth is a primal one. It has to do with instinctive responses like reproduction and the release of bodily fluids, but we've been taught to do these things privately as humans.

33

Stop!' Our new brain, along with cultural and social conditioning, can often get in the way of birth. This is something you can't do in front of him/her.'

Analyzes is another task that your new brain engages in. You apply insights from the past, as well as what you've already learned, to what could happen in the future. You do this by bringing a variety of possibilities into the present, which can affect how you behave and make decisions at that moment.

This is a very disabling element for humans when it comes to birth, and it gets in the way. Other mammals benefit from the fact that their bodies go about their business without them having to wonder, "Is that normal?" "What does that mean?" "Would what happened to my friend happen to me?"

Your inner narrator goes to sleep when you do. Close your eyes and consider what you'll need in your room before going to bed. Make a list of everything you want to do. It may be necessary for it to be dark, clean, and quiet; you may prefer it to be warm or cold.

Your doors will be locked, and your curtains or blinds will most likely be drawn. This is the kind of place where your inner narrator likes to unwind. It can be more difficult to silence the inner narrator and fall asleep if you are thinking a lot and have something on your mind.

You are teaching your neo-cortex to calm down with the strategies you are learning. While you get into your birthing zone and your body spontaneously births your infant, you're learning how to lull your inner narrator to sleep and relax.

THE THREE FUNDAMENTAL METHODOLOGIES

Staying in your birthing zone and keeping the inner narrator at bay can be accomplished in three easy measures. Every visualization or other hypnosis technique in this book is built on these foundations.

To stay in contact with your body, focused, and solid, you'll need to learn to be mindfully present in your birthing zone.

The **first step** is to build your birth mantra by tuning into the rhythm of your breath. A mantra is a meaningful phrase repeated with each breath, such as "breathe in, relax, breathe out, let go." Staying mindfully with your breath might be all you need; many women report that once they've practiced this on a regular basis, it's very easy to remain rooted in the birthing region.

Step 2 deepens your relaxation by causing your muscles to relax. This is often referred to as a 'rapid relaxation.'

When you progress to **Step 3**, you will be in a much deeper state of hypnosis, blocking out external distractions and focusing solely on yourself. This is referred to as a "conditioned relaxation." This is a basic but effective technique that your birth partner will learn once it has been conditioned by practice.

Follow the first three measures outlined below before beginning any of the visualizations or other activities in the book. In addition to listening to your hypnosis songs, you can practice these methods for at least 10 minutes a day. Find a quiet place to relax and listen to the Mindful Hypnobirthing instrumental hypnosis track in the background. Setting a timer for five minutes can be beneficial.

Then, as you become more comfortable with it and notice that the timer is going off too fast, train yourself to extend the duration to 10 minutes, 15 minutes, or even longer if desired.

STEP 1: EXERCISE MINDFULLY

You breathe without thought every day, but how often do you sit quietly and focus on your breath? When you concentrate on your breathing during pregnancy or labour, your focus changes inwards and away from any things in your world that could make you feel uneasy or take you out of your birthing zone. Some people find it difficult to keep their minds from wandering at first, and they complain, "I can't help worrying about other things." It's called a practice because the more you do it, the better it gets. You'll discover that you can find a stillness that allows you to bond with your body and your baby without the distractions of everyday life. Your brain can't concentrate on something else when it's concentrating on anything like your breath.

At any given moment, your conscious mind can only retain a small amount of knowledge. When it comes to giving birth, this is a fantastic ability to have. It's an easy and efficient strategy to use your breath to hold you in your birthing region.

1. Make sure you're breathing deeply from your abdomen to begin. Place one hand on your chest and the other on your stomach. Close your eyes and note which hand moves faster than the other. When the hand on your chest moves, take deeper breaths until your belly feels like it's breathing in and out, and the hand on your belly moves more.

2. Breathe in for a count of six and out for a count of eight. A 'lengthening breath' occurs when your out-breath is longer than your in-breath. If you've been doing pregnancy yoga, you're probably familiar with this as the golden thread. Alternatively, you may prefer to simply breathe slowly in and out, noticing the warmth of the air and the movement of your breath down into your body and out again. When practicing your birth breath, the most important thing is to get into a relaxed and familiar rhythm. After the out-breath, you'll notice that you'll naturally pause for one to three seconds before taking another breath.

3. You can find that you get wrapped up in daily thoughts and emotions when you learn to quiet your mind and follow your breath. This is to be expected when you first begin practicing. When you notice yourself doing this, bring your attention back to your breathing and repeat to yourself, "Breathing in and breathing out." Allow

yourself to let go of any preconceived notions that you can't do it because you can; all it takes is a regular practice.

STEP 2: RELAX, RELAX, RELAX, RELAX, RELAX, RELAX, RELAX, RELAX, RELAX, RELAX, RELAX

You will start to relax your muscles even further once you've relaxed into your breathing and found a good pattern of breathing in and breathing out. This light hypnosis exercise is designed to help you relax quickly. You can train your body to respond to this command by letting go and relaxing your muscles quickly and easily. This is a fantastic technique that can be applied to a variety of situations in life, such as making a presentation, participating in sports, or preparing for an exam. You can apply it to whatever you like for the rest of your life once you've learned it.

Imagine yourself outside, in a place where you are at ease, relaxed, and warm. Recognize the warmth of the sun on your head, which causes your hair to feel wet.

3. Enable the warmth from your head and chest to move down your body.

2. Allowing the abdomen and pelvis to relax deeply is step two.

1. Now, stretch your calves and ankles all the way down to your knees and toes.

Then repeat after me: "Relax, relax, relax."

You just follow the rhythm once you've gotten used to this ease in your body and it's well-conditioned:

Breathe in, 'Three, two, one,' breathe out, 'Relax, relax, relax, and your muscles will automatically let go of any tension This will assist you in gaining a sense of self-awareness and tuning in to your body.

HYPNOSIS DEEPENER (STEP 3)

A hypnosis deepener is a device that allows you to enter a more comfortable state of hypnosis. You'll learn it in a very straightforward manner that you can either do yourself or teach to your partner. After you've developed a breathing pattern and practiced breathing in 'three, two, one,' and breathing out, 'relax, relax, relax,' slowly count down from ten to one in your mind.

Steps 1, 2, and 3 will help you get used to being in your birthing environment. It's perfectly fine if you choose one over the other. You may use either the quick calming or the breathing and deepener on your own. Remember to personalize it; what works for you is what you should do. If you can, practice the deepener with your partner; having your birth partner feel secure with these basic foundation strategies before the birth can help.

CHAPTER FIVE

LETTING GO OF FEAR AND ANXIETY

When it comes to birth, the body and mind are inextricably linked. From the moment you are born until now, your own life experiences and values will cause unconscious physical responses in your body, often overpowering what you actively want to feel.

We'll discuss why pain can be caused by fear and anticipation of pain in this chapter. Understanding how your brain might obstruct a positive birth experience can assist you in identifying and releasing your doubts about birth. As a result, you build the space inside yourself to allow your body to birth naturally without the tension and anxiety that fear can bring. You'll have answered and let go of any concerns by the end of this chapter, laying the groundwork for new optimistic beliefs.

THE PERFECT MACHINE THAT IS YOUR BODY

Do you have a thorough understanding of how the body functions during labour? Most adolescent girls receive very little sex education and grow up with little understanding of their bodies and what happens to them during childbirth.

Have you ever considered how your body creates a complex human being from a single egg and sperm? Without your brain thinking about it, your body will build a heart, lungs, eyes, and kidneys during the nine months you are pregnant. That's fantastic. Scientists have spent years attempting to create artificial organs, but you have done so without even realizing it.

Your fist-sized womb will expand to make room for your growing baby and their tiny world. During pregnancy, the body goes through a lot of changes, but most women embrace them and don't let them bother them. You can experience niggles and tweaks as your internal organs migrate, with your heart and lungs moving higher to make room for your growing baby. You may have a pinched nerve here and there, as well as back pain and signs that your ligaments are softening.

So, while you may understand that your tissues expand and soften during pregnancy to accommodate an infant, how do you feel about birth? Do you think your body is capable of completing the task? Are you concerned about how you'll get 'that out of there,' as many women in my classes say? If you believe this, note that it is not your body's fault; it is the inability of others to educate you about birth anatomy. Your body is designed to nurture and develop a human baby, and it is also designed to give birth to your baby in a way that is ideal for both of you. If women could conceive but not give birth, evolution would be severely hampered. The problem is that being afraid of birth, whatever your fear is, causes changes in your body that can slow down labour, make it more painful and difficult, or even stop it entirely.

HORMONES THAT ARE BENEFICIAL

To comprehend how fear affects your body, you must first comprehend the role of hormones in the initiation and termination of labour. Your hormones are the most responsive component of your birthing body, and the way you think, both consciously and unconsciously, communicates with them, slowing or speeding up labour.

Let's pretend that you consider birth to be a routine occurrence. You were raised in a culture that values life, where women are blessed and cared for with love during childbirth, and where women look forward to giving birth to their children. Because of this help and knowledge, you will relax and trust your body as it softens and expands during birth, just as it does during pregnancy. When this occurs, the body produces a large amount of the birth hormone oxytocin.

OXYTOCIN

Oxytocin is a hormone that promotes social interaction and is the glue that keeps our societies together. We are a vulnerable species that would not thrive in the wild against more powerful predators if we were left alone, so being in groups and societies keeps us safe and protected. Even today, studies show that being a member of a group, feeling loved and linked, lowers the risk of certain illnesses, including heart disease. Your limbic brain, or old part of your brain, is where you get your sense of culture and attachment. It is focused on your experiences in the womb, at birth, and in your early years by identifying relationships with your parents and others in your immediate environment.

Oxytocin also aids in the development of our children. We usually only have one child at a time. We must properly care for them by nurturing love in order for them to live and prosper. This is a unique evolutionary technique that distinguishes mammals from other species and is aided by Oxytocin.

Oxytocin, also known as the love hormone, promotes reproduction by making sex enjoyable. It also encourages women to want to have children. During pregnancy, women who are fearless have free-flowing Oxytocin. Their birth stories are frequently much more optimistic and self-affirming than many of the ones you see on TV today.

BETA-ENDORPHINS

Beta-endorphins are generated in response to the uninterrupted release of Oxytocin. These are the natural painkillers and feel-good hormones generated by your body. They can only be made from naturally occurring Oxytocin, not synthetic Oxytocin.

Beta-endorphins are a natural blessing that allows women to have a strong and euphoric birthing experience. Many women I've met have expressed their desire to do it again and again; this is how birth should be. I'm not referring to a painless birth; rather, I'm referring to a birth that is free of misery and full of control. There is a minor distinction.

YOUR BABY WAS CREATED TO BE LOVED BY

You Oxytocin's bonding properties often suggest that your baby was created to be loved and cared for by you. We give birth to our babies at a very young age, and they are completely reliant on their mothers for survival. The rush of Oxytocin is the rush of love we experience when our babies are born, and it binds us to them. Your love for your child will shield them from harm.

The benefits of Oxytocin include:

- Lowering your pulse rate and blood pressure;
- Reducing any sensation of pain in your body;
- Accelerating growth and wound healing;
- Stimulating the release of prolactin for milk production;
- Supporting attachment between you and your baby;
- Triggering positive responses in the father who bonds with his baby with an Equiv.

PRIVATE HORMONE

Oxytocin is also known as the shy hormone or our private hormone. You must feel comfortable and private in order to release Oxytocin.

The most important message a woman should receive about birth, according to Sarah Buckley, a doctor who specializes in birth hormones, is that she should feel "private, protected, and unobserved." This may also refer to anyone being present but not actually staring you down. Knitting was once a common job for midwives to do during births. The sound of needles served as a reassuring reminder from the midwife that "I am here for you, but not watching you." This expertise is being reintroduced in some parts of the UK.

STRESS HORMONES AND ADRENALINE

In contrast, during the early stages of labour, adrenaline and nor-adrenaline are unwelcome guests. Adrenaline and nor-adrenaline are stress hormones that stimulate your sympathetic nervous system to help you get out of danger quickly when you feel threatened, concerned, or think you're in danger.

Blood rushes to your arms and legs, preparing you to fight or flee. When animals are endangered, they always freeze; it's the equivalent of playing dead when there's nowhere to run. It's a precautionary measure.

Adrenaline and nor-adrenaline play a vital role in helping the baby prepare physically for life outside the womb during the final stages of childbirth. It's important to understand, though, how too much adrenaline or nor-adrenaline early in labour will slow down labour and prevent the body from doing what it's supposed to do.

HOW FEAR CAN DELAY CHILDBIRTH

Four out of every five women are worried about giving birth. Who wouldn't be worried if they had to grit their teeth and get on with it? Why wouldn't you be scared if you're told that birth is "the worst pain you'll ever have," that you should "take any medication provided," and that "the only reason we do it again is that we're made to forget the pain"?

True, birth is intense and strong, and it can feel daunting at times, but not all women who give birth consider it painful. Some women enjoy it and find it to be much less difficult than they had been led to believe. Some women also have an orgasmic birth – note, Oxytocin is the sex hormone, and when your body is filled with Oxytocin, your body is primed for an ecstatic experience.

Oxytocin can flow freely in a birth that is free of fear and in which you feel safe and private. Your body sends a signal to your brain to produce more Oxytocin with each contraction, and more Oxytocin means more contractions. A positive feedback loop is what this is known as. It's as if your brain and your womb are having a private, whispered conversation that directs your body. This conversation loop assists you in releasing all of the hormones required for your contractions to occur and labour to progress.

Fear and anxiety have the opposite effect: they trigger the release of adrenaline and nor-adrenaline, which can slow down labour. You can't have both Oxytocin and adrenaline because they're antagonists. It's similar to a seesaw effect. The more Oxytocin you have, the less adrenaline you have; and vice versa, the more adrenaline you have, the less Oxytocin you have. As oxytocin levels drop, signals to the womb slow down, potentially slowing contractions.

EXPECTATION, ANXIETY, FEAR, AND PAIN

The anticipation of pain has two effects on our birth experience. First, anticipation can cause anxiety, which causes the body to release adrenaline and tense up. The anticipation of a painful sensation, on the other hand, may cause a painful sensation.

You are not allowed to talk about pain in certain hypnobirthing programs because talking about pain is a suggestion that draws our attention to it.

When it comes to pain and labour, if the suggestion is that there will be pain, we can begin to build an expectation and a very real perception of pain if we dwell on it.

Scientists are fascinated by pain because it is so closely linked to both perception and expectation. If we're told to anticipate pain, we'll feel it even if there isn't any. Anxiety about pain has been shown in several studies in recent years to increase both pain perceptions and pain unpleasantness. One of the most intriguing is a 2011 study from Oxford University's Professor Irene Tracey, which demonstrated how our expectation of pain could cause more pain, even overpowering powerful painkillers. Tracey's team applied heat to 22 patients' legs and asked them to rate their discomfort on a scale of 1 to 100. Those patients were hooked up to an intravenous drip so that medications could be given to them discreetly. The average pain level at the start was 66. The pain score was then reduced to 55 after patients were given a powerful painkiller without their knowledge. They were then informed that they would be given a painkiller, and their score dropped to 39. The patients were then advised that the painkiller had been removed and that they could anticipate pain without changing their dosage. Despite the fact that the powerful painkiller was still being administered, the score increased to 64, which was similar to the original measure of pain. Magnetic resonance imaging, the revealed which parts of the brain were active during the experiment, backed up the findings.

You may be afraid because you're expecting pain, which you've heard about from others. This can trigger anxiety about how you will cope, as well as a negative perception of the specific sensations of birth. When you go into labour, and your body reacts to those strange stimuli, your brain makes a quick assessment based on what you know and what you've been told. Your brain will measure labour +

unknown strong feeling = severe pain if you've been told it's a pain. Pain implies a feeling that something is wrong, and it causes stress and anxiety, which can aggravate the pain.

PAIN AND TENSION

Our bodies create stress when we are nervous or scared, and tension causes pain. The 'Fear Tension Pain Cycle' is a term used to describe this phenomenon. People who are nervous are more vulnerable to pain, both chronic and temporary, according to studies conducted by Irene Tracey's team of neuroscientists.

If you have lower levels of anxiety, the body will be able to cope with any physical sensations more effectively, and any discomfort you experience will be significantly reduced. Birth may be totally painless for certain women.

People who have had a pain-free birth experience describe it as a powerful, intense feeling rather than pain. Many second-time mothers attend my class because they are confident in their ability to deliver a healthy baby and are looking for strategies to help them concentrate. Most second births are quicker than first births, not only because the mother's body has already given birth to a child but also because the mother knows deep down that she can do it and knows what to expect. As she approaches the birth of her infant, a first-time mother may be filled with anxiety from all the stories she's heard and a sense of the unknown, causing tension and apprehension.

HOW DOES TENSION AFFECT YOUR PREGNANCY BODY?

Understanding how apprehension and stress affect the birthing body is important. There are three sets of muscles in your uterus, and we'll concentrate on the two most essential for relaxed contractions:

1. Longitudinal: These are like fingers that run lengthwise and open the lower circular muscles with each contraction.

2. Lower Circular: When the cervix opens, the longitudinal muscles gently draw these muscles up along the circumference of the uterus.

These muscle groups work together to soften and loosen your cervix. They're just like any other group of muscles in your body that work together, such as your biceps and triceps when lifting a shopping bag or the interplay of muscles when swallowing; they're built to work together so that your body can do what it needs to do at the time. They cluster at the top of the uterus as they contract and withdraw, adding thickness and strength to drive your baby down and out when your body is ready. It's an incredibly well-coordinated and clever birthing body feature.

If you're nervous or scared of giving birth, your muscles will contract because they don't want you to give birth in a place where you feel threatened or unsafe. Instead, they firm up to keep the baby from going down. You wait if you need to use the restroom and there is nowhere to go that is private, don't you?

Birth follows the same privacy and safety laws, and the more comfortable you are, the easier it is for these muscles to relax and do their job.

When things slow down or stop, the first medical reaction could be to 'look for something wrong' rather than to consider 'what has changed?' 'Is the mother at ease?' 'Does she feel secure?' If medications are used to speed up labour at this stage, it simply means that the stressed muscles are being forced to do something they don't want to do. This is why many women experience discomfort.

The pelvic region is, of course, connected to your leg muscles. The muscles that supply blood to your legs so you can run away run down through the psoas muscles in your back when you're in fight or flight mode. The pelvic region is also traversed by these muscles. Because of the increased blood flow, certain muscles become firmer and larger when you are tense. Pumping your biceps is the perfect way to feel this! Isn't there a difference between the muscle when it's soft and when it's hard?

When you're free of fear and instead optimistic, comfortable, and calm, all of these muscles relax, which means there's more room in the pelvis for the baby to move down and gain from every millimetre of your pelvic space.

WHAT IS THE SOURCE OF FEAR?

Fear can stem from a variety of sources: the physical changes that occur during labour, the suffering that other women have described, or the hospital and procedures themselves. It may also be minor concerns such as if you will arrive at the hospital on time, whether you will have childcare for your children, or if your husband will return if he works a long-distance away.

There may be persistent suggestions that something is wrong and that you are endangering your child. Your visits to the midwife during pregnancy are made up of tests and checks on the infant. Some are essential, but others can instill fear where none should exist. Any test you take requires you to meet a norm, an average, from which any deviation can be interpreted as cause for concern or further investigation.

MAKING A BLANK CANVAS FOR YOUR BABY'S BIRTH

You might think, "I've got it!" until you've grasped the idea. 'I know what I should do.' This is, however, where hypnosis training varies from other types of mental preparation. What you think you know might not be the same as what is subconsciously processed.

An involuntary and instinctive fear response can overpower your conscious thoughts and activate automatic responses in your body, activated by what your unconscious believes it knows. This is especially true in circumstances where you are apprehensive or nervous without even realizing it. Hypnosis is all about reprogramming your automatic responses so that they unconsciously comply with the healthy optimistic desires, intentions, and values that you have in your conscious consciousness.

This is a crucial part of figuring out how hypnobirthing can work for you. The best way to explain how the relationship between the two parts of your brain functions is to illustrate how a phobia grows over time but can be resolved in a matter of hours. A phobia is a fear-based reflex reaction caused by something that makes you anxious. Understanding how a phobia develops will help you comprehend that resetting your entire mind is critical if you want a gentle birth.

Think about it now if you have a phobia or a fear of something, put yourself in that situation, knowing you are safe where you are, and allow yourself to feel the emotion associated with that fear. Any of the signs that your sympathetic nervous system has been stimulated may be obvious to you: your heart may be pounding a little faster, your breathing may be faster, and your palms may be sweaty.

As humans, our survival response has become a little muddled as a result of the mixed signals we receive from the moment we are born until now. Phobias are the product of this, and they are an unconscious survival response in situations where we don't need to be in survival mode.

Things people have seen or heard in films, on television, online, or in the news can cause phobias. Phobias and anxieties are fascinating because they are a natural reaction to something that will not hurt them. People with phobias are acutely aware of this and sometimes feel foolish for behaving in this way, but they are unable to stop themselves. Phobias may also prevent people from doing something they want to do, such as travelling or riding an escalator.

The good news is that you can quickly overcome a phobia or fear – it's like hitting the reset button.

HOW TO RESET YOUR BIRTH BRAIN?

Consider the brain as a map, with neurons linking various parts of the brain like roads leading to different destinations on a map. Your map is one-of-a-kind, and the routes and destinations change over time as you gain new experiences. Your brain was already setting down paths, destinations, and pathways on your own unique map when you were born, all of which have an effect on how you react to your environment in your own unique way. This brain mapping occurs at a rapid rate between birth and the age of three, then slows down but continues to be very quick until about the age of thirteen. Much of our automatic responses to the world around us are created during this period, and we are at our most impressionable.

This capacity to alter pathways in your brain, known as 'brain plasticity,' lasts well into old age. The good news is that you can still alter your paths, destinations, and pathways in relation to any circumstance or destination, including your reactions to birth. Resetting your birth brain literally entails creating new neural pathways and altering your reference system so that the path you take to birth is different and better. While it may have taken years to develop a fear, anxiety, or phobia, it can be reset in as little as an hour.

CHAPTER SIX

CREATING POSITIVE BIRTH BELIEFS

Y ou've overcome your anxiety and built a blank canvas on which to rewrite your birth story. From this point forward, you must ensure that the messages you receive, both from yourself and others, convey a positive birth message and are compatible with the type of birth you want.

This can be accomplished in three ways:

1. Understanding how internal signals shape beliefs that can support or impede your birth, as well as how to alter them.

2. Recognizing how you absorb knowledge from your surroundings.

3. Adding safe, optimistic birth photos to your birth reference system.

Would your internal beliefs work against you or for you?

Take some time to consider the kind of birth you want to have. Are your convictions supportive of that aim and compatible with the type of birth you desire? Examine your heart: do you believe you can have a meaningful and inspiring birth experience? Do you think your body is capable of completing the task? Do you think you have a say in the matter? Do you think your child is the right size for your body? Do you think birth is a regular, natural occurrence rather than a medical one?

What we believe will become a self-fulfilling prophecy. Action forms belief, and knowledge shapes belief.

Your views can be either negative or positive. They can come from a place of love and acceptance, or they can come from a place of fear. The way you think about pregnancy will influence how you feel about being pregnant and giving birth. If your values favour conscientious hypnobirthing, your experience will most likely be more positive; if they don't, you're posing obstacles to your hypnobirthing target and casting doubt on your ability to achieve it. This interpretation of how our internal belief systems function has been tested in a number of studies and is referred to as "selective attention" or the "cocktail party effect" in scientific circles.

If you go to a crowded and noisy party, you could be standing there talking with someone when you hear a friend's name or a place of work mentioned by someone nearby. The knowledge is picked up by your brain in the midst of all the noise. You may be thinking, "What a coincidence!" In reality, like a filter, your brain is constantly processing and deleting information. Before it entered your conscious awareness, any information that was meaningless to you was already filtered out.

BELIEVE THAT BIRTH CAN BE A WONDERFUL EXPERIENCE.

Changing the way you think of birth is the key to developing a positive belief. If you've done so, you'll be able to alter the messages you get about birth, both subconsciously and consciously. When you have a positive conviction, the brain will look for evidence to support that belief. Consider it like' resetting your filter.' Suddenly, you'll see more tales of wonderful births, blogs, memes, tv programs, empowering encounters, and opportunities to share hints and advice about uncomplicated birth and less about trauma.

To change a belief, you must first take deliberate action to change it before it becomes a habitual part of your birth planning. The external messages you receive and the internal messages you send yourself must both help the aim of hypnobirthing with mindfulness.

EXTERNAL MESSAGES CHANGING

Changing the messages you receive from your external world is more difficult than changing your internal values, but taking practical action to change the input you receive is easier than you would expect. Of course, you can't manage anything in your world, but you can reframe the things you can. Simply put, reframing is the process of changing a negative thought into a constructive one. If something upsets you or makes you doubt your ability to give birth, ask yourself these questions to turn negative signals into constructive ones:

1. From whose point of view and based on what evidence?
2. What aspects of this experience would be beneficial to me? What can I gain from this experience?
3. In this case, what will I say to a close friend?
4. What would I do right now if I were doing the conscious hypnobirthing that I know I'm capable of?

When witnessing other people's perspectives, having a sense of perspective is crucial. Midwives also state that they will see what they consider to be a wonderful birth, while the mother will consider it to be a disaster. Another woman, on the other hand, may have had a difficult birth, according to a midwife, but she would have had a very positive experience, in fact.

Take a step back and note that much of the knowledge you're given is based on your own beliefs and perspectives. Allow yourself the freedom to alter your views and perceptions of birth as it is presented to you.

FIVE SIMPLE STEPS TO SENDING POSITIVE MESSAGES

1. CHANGE THE BOOKS THAT YOU READ

There are several pregnancy books online. Among the more general pregnancy books, there are those that motivate women by teaching them about their bodies and birth. Take the time to look for books that can provide you with the messages you need to hear and that are in line with your objectives. Read a book that teaches you about your incredible body, gives you the ability to trust it, and encourages you to be patient during labour.

2. QUIT WATCHING ADRENALINE-FUELED BIRTHS ON TV.

Many shows feature women giving birth. Remember that these will be edited, so consider your point of view and detail. We don't really have all of the truth about what we're watching. Perhaps the editor's views are reflected in an edited show. Rather than showing gentle, quiet births, producers of famous documentaries and authors of television shows often want dramatic, attention-getting storylines. The understanding of birth can be skewed by watching births on television. If you want to see a birth that is compatible with mindful hypnobirthing, ask a friend to find some for you on YouTube, or look for a Facebook page or blog that shares positive stories on a regular basis.

3. LOOK FOR POSITIVE ONLINE FORUMS

Some online forums are hotbeds of potential disasters. Look for a hypnobirthing support group on the internet. There are a plethora of options available. These forums will provide information about positive births, and being around people who support your birth decisions is often beneficial.

4. CHOOSE THE BIRTH STORIES YOU WOULD LIKE TO HEAR.

When you're eight months pregnant, instead of listening to a colleague's painful birth story, you might say, "I just don't need to hear this right now." It's common to find that women who have had regular, meaningful experiences don't talk about them much. "I didn't want to be arrogant because everyone around me seemed to have such bad stories to share," several women claim. If you have a friend who has had a relatively simple birth, inquire about it!

5. PARTICIPATE IN A POSITIVE BIRTH CLASS

Yoga, active birth, doula-led classes, relaxation, and hypnosis are only a few of the classes that help women prepare for an uncomplicated birth. If they know the emphasis will be on pain and intervention, some women prefer not to attend classes. It's not unusual for certain more traditional classes to also show you forceps or an epidural needle, which will, of course, expose you to the suggestion and belief in medical intervention.

You'll also meet other pregnant women who are looking for a similar experience to you, which will be extremely beneficial in terms of encouraging you along your path. Look for a supportive birth community near you if you can't afford a class or don't have the time. These groups have sprung up all over the world and hold daily meetings to assist women in getting a healthy birth experience. They are frequently well-resourced, with books, videos, and knowledge that can help to reinforce a healthy belief that you are designed to give birth to your child and that you can do it safely and enjoy the process.

INTERNAL MESSAGES CHANGING

Internal messaging's first concept is to "be kind to yourself" and to be your own closest birth mate. Stopping the cycle of negative thought that allows fears to develop again is the goal of changing a belief. Encourage yourself by gently reminding yourself that you can do it; your body is built to give birth, and women all over the world do it successfully every day. One of those women, maybe you.

AFFIRMATIONS FOR BIRTH

Another way to change your views is to use affirmations to change the messages you send yourself about birth. I've written a few examples below; change them up to make them sound like something you'd say, then type them out yourself to take ownership of them. Place them in a prominent location in your home or at work so that you can see them on a regular basis. Say them at least twice a day.

If you have a doubt that keeps repeating itself in your mind, write an affirmation that counteracts it. If you're worried about tearing during labour, write something like, "As I relax and let go, following my breath, my body gently expands, allowing the perfect-sized room for my baby to move through." Make certain that each affirmation is a good one.

POSITIVE AFFIRMATIONS FOR YOU

1. I am aware that my body is well constructed to carry my child into the world.
2. I believe in my birth instincts and pay attention to them.
3. As my body changes, I relish each new development, knowing that my body is constructing the ideal temporary home for my baby.
4. The closer my baby's due date approaches, the more relaxed I am.

5. It's easier for me to feel secure and in control when I'm relaxed.
6. When I go into labour, I'll fall into my routine quickly and comfortably.
7. I'm certain that I'll know when it's the right time to go to the hospital/call the midwife.
8. I'll become more comfortable with each contraction wave.
9. As I anticipate the birth of my child, I am both excited and calm.
10. I understand that during labour, my body is built to soften and expand.
11. My body will loosen and grow the more I relax.
12. The more I soften and stretch, the faster my baby can arrive in the world.
13. With each contraction wave, my baby gets closer to being born.
14. Labour is difficult, but I am certain that I am capable of completing it.
15. I'm looking forward to seeing my baby for the first time.
16. I am confident in my ability to be a wonderful mother. Make your own.

Affirmations may be beneficial to the birth partner as well. Invite them to participate in writing your affirmations with you and discussing how you want to experience your birth.

YOUR BIRTH PARTNER'S AFFIRMATIONS

These can also aid in the development of the birth partner's faith, not just as a birth partner but also in believing that mum knows what she's doing.

1. I am a caring, gentle, and compassionate birth companion.
2. I am in awe of how nature works as my partner and our baby develop.

3. I have faith that when labour starts, my partner will instinctively know what to do.
4. I'll give her the freedom to act on her instincts.
5. I will be calm, patient, and caring.
6. I'll be mindful of my own concerns and put them aside until after the birth.
7. I will be solid, still, and relaxed with my partner during each contraction wave.
8. I'll feel comfortable telling the midwife about our expectations.
9. I'm looking forward to meeting my child and becoming a dad. Make your own.

Relax and let Hypnotic Suggestion do the work for you.

Every day, as instructed in the previous chapter's Practice Guidelines, listen to your hypnosis tracks.

Suggestions are often overt and sometimes subtle, but they are both structured in a way that encourages you to embrace and own those values unconsciously. At the end of the day, it is up to you to let those convictions take hold. Since you're reading this book, and your goal is to improve your thinking so you can change your birth experience, you'll be able to make these adjustments quickly and easily. This is done in such a subtle way that you might not even notice the changes. You can simply feel lighter, healthier, and peacefully anticipating the birth of your child.

CHAPTER SEVEN

HYPNOBIRTHING TOOL KIT

It's time to learn how to use the incredible and life-changing hypnobirthing toolkit. In this chapter, you'll learn two breathing exercises (both game-changers), some visualizations, light-touch massage, directed relaxations, optimistic affirmations, and the art of creating relaxation shortcuts. Take pleasure in it. And take a deep breath.

The most important thing you will do during labour is to breathe. If you just remember one thing from this novel, make it this!

A successful breathing technique benefits you in many ways. For starters, it means that you are getting enough oxygen into your bloodstream, which your muscles need to function properly. You wouldn't attempt to exercise while gasping for air. The same can be said for labour and delivery. Second, sticking to a breathing strategy keeps you calm and prevents panic breathing/hyperventilation. Finally, concentrating on your breath during each surge diverts your attention away from the feeling you're having, making each surge more manageable. Rather than getting caught up in the waves and feeling out of control, you can stay calm and grounded by focusing on your breath.

Counting along with your breathing technique or visualizations can be extremely beneficial in keeping you on track.

You will learn two very basic and easy breathing techniques in this chapter. These alone would improve the quality of your work. I suggest that you put them into practice as much as possible so that they become second nature. The first breathing technique is known as 'up breathing.' It is a lovely relaxing breath that you can use during the day to help you relax. A few rounds of this breath before bed will almost certainly assist you in falling asleep. The other breathing technique, known as 'down breathing,' is excellent for going to the bathroom. As a result, the bathroom is an excellent place to do this! You'll find a practice schedule at the back of this book that you can use if you like. It's up to you how much you practice, but the more you do, the more powerful all of these methods and strategies can become.

Up breathing, to keep it easy, is used during the 'up stage' of labour, when the muscles contract and the cervix opens. The 'down stage' of labour is when the muscles begin to shift downwards, slowly pushing the baby out.

The first thing I want to tell you about is that you will know when you've reached the downstage, and it's time to change your breathing style because you will feel your body start to push and your baby move down the birth canal; it's an unmistakable feeling. If you're a first-time mother-to-be or not, believe me when I say you'll know. It's similar to pooping. How do you know when it's time to leave? You don't wait until the poop is halfway out to go to the bathroom. You normally feel a sense of pressure coming on, and you just know.

The second thing I want you to know is that you don't have to be concerned about what could happen if you forget to turn and continue to breathe up throughout the downstage of labour. The answer is that nothing negative will occur. It's perfectly good if you prefer to breathe in for four seconds and out for eight during your entire labour and delivery; the most important thing is that you keep breathing! You're doing an excellent job if you're taking in oxygen and breathing out rather than tensing and holding your breath. It'll be a lot more relaxed.

However, you can find that as your body begins to drive, it becomes more difficult to maintain your up breathing. Slowly inhale and feel your chest rise and expand as your uterus muscles press back in the opposite direction is difficult. When you exhale, you will find that you begin to make a mooing sound as your body powerfully moves downwards involuntarily. This is perfectly natural and perfectly fine; it could simply mean that it's time to turn to down breathing, which will be much easier at this stage.

UP BREATHING

This is the most critical to learn because you'll be doing it for the longest period of time. Nobody can predict how long the labour will last, but the first stage, the 'up stage,' when the uterus muscles contract and the cervix soften and open to completely dilated, usually lasts longer than the second stage, the 'down stage,' when the uterus muscles reverse direction and force the baby down the birth canal and into the big wide world. This stage will last anywhere from a few minutes to several hours, while the first stage would most likely take several hours (although, of course, not always).

The good news is that up breathing is simple to do and feels great, so it's a breath you'll probably want to practice.

It's also worth noting that this breathing method isn't unique to hypnobirthing. It is used to support people with insomnia and anxiety, as well as in mindfulness practices. It works because it lowers your heart rate and makes you relax; it's an ability you can use for the rest of your life.

So, let's go for it!

Make sure you're sitting in a comfortable place. Close your eyes for a moment and block out what's going on around you. Then slowly count to four when inhaling deeply through your nose and filling your lungs. Then, when counting to eight, slowly exhale through your mouth, allowing the air to slowly move through your lips.

Exhaling for eight counts can be difficult at first, particularly while pregnant, because the baby prevents your lungs from fully filling.

However, with practice, it will become easier, and you will notice that when you're in labour and your baby moves further into your pelvis, you'll be able to breathe more easily. If you're having trouble, try exhaling for six counts instead. Simply make your exhale longer than your inhale to achieve a soothing and relaxing effect. This breathing strategy is the polar opposite of panic breathing or hyperventilating, in which the inhale rate increases while the exhale rate decreases to almost non-existent. The result we want to achieve is the polar opposite.

Let's give it a shot right now.

Inhale 2, 3, 4, and exhale 2, 3, 4, 5, 6, 7, 8.

Do the same thing again, but this time with four breath repetitions. So four times over, in for four and out for eight. If you're with somebody, make them count for you.

You should now be feeling nice and comfortable. It's normal to feel a little dizzy. The more you practice this breath, the more you'll feel like you're floating on a cloud. It has a similar feel to natural gas and air, and most people enjoy it.

The significance of repeating the up breathing four times is important. It takes about 48 seconds to do four repetitions of the up breathing technique. When you're in developed labour, this is how long a surge or contraction usually lasts. Imagine a surge (contraction) steadily rising to a peak of strength, then easing off and releasing until you feel nothing at all; after four repetitions, the surge will have either passed entirely or, at the very least, be on the release – you will have passed the peak.

Surges can be thought of in this way, and breaking them down helps to make labour more manageable. Many women have heard tales of lasting labour hours and believe that once labour begins, it will be one long contraction before the baby is born. In fact, you will feel a surge that lasts about 45 seconds to a minute, followed by a brief break of a few minutes and then another surge. This is the typical pattern of proven labour: three surges in a ten-minute cycle, each lasting approximately 45 seconds. This pattern can last for several hours, but it is much easier to manage when broken down in this way and dealt with a surge by surge.

Milli Hill once estimated that a woman only feels something during normal labour for around 23% of the time. She doesn't have any interactions the remaining 77% of the time. So, even though your labour lasts ten hours, you will only be feeling labour pains for just over two hours.

Every surge takes you closer to your son, says the affirmation. There are no surges that aren't used. Close your eyes and begin to inhale, counting to four, then slowly exhale and count to eight. Do this four times, and the wave will have passed by the time you're done, and you'll know you're one step closer to meeting your son.

Inhale calm and exhale stress is another favorite affirmation. As you inhale for four counts, imagine your body expanding and overflowing with relaxation, and then as you exhale for eight counts, imagine all stress dissipating as your whole body softens and relaxes. I hope you enjoy practicing this breathing technique and that you will use it not only for birth but for the rest of your life while you are stressed. You have a very basic but extremely effective tool at your disposal. The best part is that you still have it with you, and it's absolutely open. You'll never forget to pack it again! Don't forget to use your oxygen because you take it with you everywhere you go.

DOWN BREATHING

Your uterus muscles will begin to push downwards at some point, and you will feel the shift in direction, followed by increasing pressure as your baby descends. Now is the time to change your breathing pattern.

This stage is less about relaxation (though relaxation is always important) and more about the activity; you are giving birth to your baby! If you imagine blowing out a candle, you won't exhale slowly, so the flame would just waver and not go out. You'd guide your breath with purpose. You'd use your breath deliberately. This is what happens when you practice down breathing: you use your breath with intention and concentration. You force your breath downwards as you exhale through your mouth to help your muscles drive your baby down and out.

When it comes to the down stage of labour, there is no counting involved. Simply inhale quickly and deeply through your nose, filling your lungs, and then exhale slowly and deeply through your mouth, channelling the out-breath down your body. Then you do it again. And you repeat this process until the surge has passed, at which point you can resume normal breathing.

Most people find up breathing to be easier to master; you inhale for four counts through your nose and exhale for eight counts through your mouth – simple as that! Down breathing without counting is, on the other hand, a bit more difficult to grasp. Here are a few pointers to assist you.

Rest your hands just above your hips, at the bottom of your ribs, while you practice down breathing. When you inhale, there will be little movement, but when you exhale with concentration and purpose, channelling your breath downwards, your muscles can react and almost push downwards with your breath. Experiment with it a few times. You've cracked it if you can feel the muscles moving downwards as you breathe. During the down stage of labour, your muscles will be powerfully pressing downwards with each surge, and by using this breath, you will ensure that you are working with rather than against your uterus muscles. You are assisting with the improvement of everything. You're not pushing; instead, you're assisting your muscles with your breath. All of the hard work will be done by the muscles.

When it comes to practice, down breathing isn't going to help you fall asleep peacefully, which is why it's always recommended that you do your practice in a specific location or when doing a specific "activity."

Yes, on the toilet when it's time to go! It's the ideal time and location to work on your down breathing. It is preferable for women to place a small sticky note on the back of their toilet door at home with the words "down breathing" written on it as a reminder. Then, once a day, when you go to the bathroom, you're ensuring daily practice. Furthermore, you're conditioning yourself to equate down breathing with relaxation and softening, as well as something being removed from the body. Yes, it's a poo, not an infant, but the feeling of increasing pressure is eerily close to the beginning of the down stage of childbirth. You may also discover that down breathing makes it easier to go to the bathroom – more breathing, less pressure! In any case, the more you practice, the more natural it will become on the big day.

When watching positive birth videos on YouTube, you might find it helpful to pay special attention near the end, just before the baby is born. Try to hear the woman in the video using her breath while she is in the down stage of labour. This will help you understand how down-breathing is used in practice.

Finally, it's normal to be concerned about how you'll know when you've reached this low point, but you'll just know. Your body will begin to push downwards, and it will be an unmistakable feeling. Many women have said that they instinctively turned to down breathing at this stage because it was more relaxed – it was not a deliberate decision.

ILLUSTRATIONS

Some people will fall in love with the breathing counting technique and will begin to rely on their birth partner to count for them, guiding them through each surge. If this works for you, that's fantastic. It's a perfect opportunity for your birth partner to be interested if you practice with them. Others may prefer the space to be silent, or they may prefer to listen to music or read relaxation books.

If counting isn't calming for you or you don't have anyone to count for you, visualization is another way to pace your breathing. Using an upward visualization to go along with your up breathing is a smart idea. Consider a hot air balloon: as you inhale, the balloon fills with air and inflates until it becomes a large circular balloon. Then imagine the hot air balloon gradually rising into the sky and floating off into the distance as you slowly exhale.

You might imagine the sun rising over the horizon as you inhale, then slowly creeping upwards to its midday location above your head as you exhale. Imagine experiencing the sun's warmth as it rises higher in the sky.

Alternatively, imagine a party balloon inflating and expanding when you inhale and then feeling all the air escape as the balloon shrinks rapidly as you exhale. Choose a color for your balloon since it will aid in visualization.

People also use opening visualizations to help with down breathing. For example, imagine all the layers of a rose bud unfolding and opening as you exhale.

Some women will use visualizations that they are already acquainted with, such as those learned in yoga classes. The 'golden thread' visualization is a common one: imagine a golden thread running from your lips and stretching out to the horizon as you exhale. Breaking your breath breaks the thread, which is a picture that could help you stick to the long exhale.

During the down stage of labour, some women imagine their baby moving down the birth canal and concentrate on the fact that they will see their baby soon. Perhaps they will imagine how their baby's face will appear, whether he or she is a boy or a girl, or how they will show their baby to siblings or other family members. Allowing yourself to be distracted by positive thoughts is enjoyable.

It's just a matter of finding something that works for you and helps you sustain the in-for-four and out-for-eight breath rhythm.

It doesn't matter what you want. Simply set aside some time per day to practice breathing while visualizing. It's best to do a few repetitions each evening before bedtime to help you relax into sleep, but you can also practice anytime you remember during the day.

You'll probably notice that you're already counting quietly in your mind while attempting to follow the visualization at first. You'll get used to the rhythm of your breath and what four and eight counts feel like after some practice, and you'll be able to pace yourself while concentrating on your visualization without counting. It's true that practice makes perfect. Even if you want to make your birth partner count for you, it's a good idea to have a backup visualization in case your birth partner needs to speak with a midwife or doctor or if you need to go to the bathroom. There's no such thing as having too many options at your disposal.

POSITIVE RECOMMENDATION

Positive reprogramming is a term used in psychology to describe the process of rewiring the brain and improving the way you think. Positive reinforcement's goal is exactly the same. Consider the latter to be more friendly and less of a piece of computer software about to be plugged in and rebooted!

Positive reinforcement is essentially the act of actively searching out positive thoughts over and over before the brain's habits are altered on a physiological level (the reprogramming element). Positive affirmations (listening to or reading positive statements) or cognitive behavioral therapy (CBT) have been shown in several studies to be successful in changing the way your brain lights up and processes knowledge in your subconscious mind. It's incredible.

Many women, as well as men, are afraid of giving birth. Undoubtedly, the media, what we see on TV, and the horror stories we hear contribute to our terror. It is possible, however, to substitute our negative associations with birth with more positive ones through positive reinforcement, and as a result, to feel more positive and confident when thinking about birth.

Positive reinforcement can be used in simple ways to transform the attitude, such as:

- Creating or purchasing a series of positive affirmation cards to display in your home so you can see and absorb positive statements on a regular basis
- Watching positive birth videos
- Reading positive birth stories
- Examining photographs of happy births

It's just as necessary to consume positivity and form new positive associations with birth as it is to shield yourself from negativity, which can only sabotage your efforts. Avoid TV shows that you know feature dramatic – and traumatic – depictions of birth, don't be sucked in by internet clickbait that you know can only lead to scary or worrying stories, avoid TV dramas or novels that might cause fear, and have the confidence to ask anyone who feel it's appropriate to share their birth trauma with you at this time to please refrain from doing so – or at the very least to waive their right to do so. In the name of politeness, try not to consume someone else's unpleasant experience because it can just affect your own.

It's best to think of a filing cabinet as a metaphor. Your mind is full of data, and the ones closest to the front are the easiest to access and extract. You want to fill your brain with optimistic files while pregnant. There may be positive birth stories, positive birth videos, or positive affirmations so that when you're in labour, your subconscious mind refers to these files for comfort. What you don't want is for your cabinet – or subconscious – to be overflowing with negative files because when you're in labour, your subconscious will rely on these files to make you feel afraid, which will slow down your labour.

So, go ahead and fill the cabinet with good files and positivity, and don't let any new negativity into your life. You've already spent your whole life making negative associations with birth. Now is the time to begin forming healthy relationships.

You may notice that your mind has wandered and that you're thinking about something that worries you or makes you feel nervous. It might be something you overheard, something that happened to a friend of a friend, something you saw on TV, or even your own prior childbirth experience. If this occurs, deliberately redirect your thoughts to something positive, such as reading a positive post, watching a positive video, scrolling through a birth photography account, or repeating your positive affirmations. The more you do this, the more likely it is that if you think about birth or anyone mentions it, a good thought will arise.

Positive reinforcement requires some effort, but it has a significant effect, and the effects are felt almost instantly, as with all of these strategies. Listening to positive affirmations or reading positive affirmation cards will help you achieve your goals. You'll feel less nervous and more optimistic about giving birth almost immediately.

BEING ABLE TO TURN OFF

Relaxation isn't something we do too much in our society. When asked what they do to relax, the majority of people would say they go for a run, read a book, go out for a beer, or watch television. We often replace a less pleasurable activity (work, for example) with a pleasurable activity (a hobby, for example) and consider this to be an example of us 'relaxing.' We're merely engaging in a different form of action, in fact. We seldom switch off the lights and take time to really unwind.

We all enjoy taking a break from the stresses and demands of the day by doing something more enjoyable. That isn't always a bad thing, and it does make you feel fine, but it isn't relief.

We want to be fully comfortable – both mentally and physically – during labour. Knowing that there is a mind-body link, it makes sense that if we can maintain a sense of balance in our minds, our bodies will be comfortable as well, making birth much easier.

We can achieve this relaxation in hypnobirthing in a variety of ways. Most of it may be unfamiliar to you at first, but with practice, it will become second nature, and you will find it easier and easier to achieve the comfortable state you desire. Since daily relaxation has so many mental and physical health benefits, it's a good skill to have for life, not just during pregnancy. Mindfulness and calming techniques are taught to young children as part of the curriculum of some classrooms. Hopefully, the next generation will grow up learning how to relax properly and understand the benefits of doing so. Even if you've never done it before, achieving a state of deep relaxation with some basic resources is pretty simple (with a little practice). That's what we'll be looking at in this chapter.

RELAXATION ACTIVITIES WITH A GUIDE

These are basically mindfulness exercises and are also known as guided meditations. They are about living in the present moment, allowing your mind to be driven by the voice of your birth partner or a video, and relaxing. It's not about being hypnotized or losing control here. You are in complete charge during a guided relaxation.

While MP3s can be very helpful, it's a good idea to try some guided relaxation exercises with your birth partner. Their voice is even better because you are already familiar with it and find it to be reassuring and comforting. Your birth partner would feel more involved if you do the practice together. Lighting a candle, spritzing the room with a scented room spray, dimming the lights – and adding something else you intend on doing when giving birth – are all good ideas. Basically, practice establishing the scene! Then get relaxed (sitting or lying down), close your eyes, and let your birth partner's voice guide you through the relaxation process.

It will seem silly the first couple of times, but with practice, it will become second nature, and you will find that you enjoy taking five minutes out of your day to do this exercise with your partner.

ESTABLISHING ANCHORS

In hypnotherapy, an anchor is actually something you closely associate with a pleasant memory. It may be a scent, a specific sound (music), a sight, a specific taste (food), or a familiar touch.

Setting anchors is also known as 'conditioning.' The popular research is known as "Pavlov's Dogs" was done in the 1890s/early 1900s and was all about this idea. Pavlov, a physicist, used a metronome to make a clicking noise and then fed his puppies. After some time, he noticed that the dogs salivated in anticipation of the food when they heard the metronome. The presence of food was no longer needed to elicit this response; the dogs had been trained to equate the sound of the metronome with their food. Pavlov demonstrated that animals, including humans, could be conditioned to react to set stimuli through repeated and reinforced association.

When it comes to hypnobirthing, you're basically doing the same thing: conditioning yourself to relax in response to those stimuli, whether they're audio, touch, or something else. You're forming positive connections between these causes and a feeling of deep relaxation now that you're pregnant. When you're in labour, your body can respond to these stimuli in kind. The stimuli will become more powerful and reliable as you practice.

STROKING THE ARM

While reading the script, your birth partner will simply stroke your arm slowly, starting at the knuckles, over the wrist, then up the arm towards the elbow. It can be a light, almost tickly stroke or a firmer stroke, depending on personal preference. You will begin to equate the arm stroking with the beautiful, deep relaxation you hopefully feel if you do this each time the script is read. Your birth partner will not have time to read the entire script during childbirth, but they can use the arm-stroking feature. This will serve as a cue for you to enter that lovely, comfortable, relaxed state. This is referred to as 'setting an anchor' by hypnotherapists. The touch is the anchor in this situation, and you equate it with the deep relaxation you felt while practicing at home, feeling protected and secure. It's similar to making a shortcut to relaxation.

It's also worth noting that this method works for something else! You could ask your birth partner to stroke your hair instead if you prefer that. It's not that the arm has special abilities, but rather that you develop a connection between an action (arm stroking) and a feeling through repetition (relaxation). You can then use the movement on its own to elicit the same sensation during labour.

THE ARM IS LOWERED.

Your birth partner should gently grasp your wrist and lift your arm a little above your lap at this stage. Lifting your arm should feel heavy if it's properly comfortable. Your birth partner will then loosen their grip on your wrist and allow your arm to fall into your lap when prompted. Your arm should be limp and heavy, dropping without resistance if you've remained comfortable. If your arm seems to float and resist gravity, it's possible you're holding onto some tension in your body and partially raising the weight of your arm. You will be motivated to really let go and release all stress by repeating this arms drop three times.

Of course, a limp, relaxed arm would not make birth any easier, but if your arm is limp and relaxed, your whole body is likely to be tension-free as well. Since there is no resistance or internal struggle, the more relaxed your muscles are in your body, the more comfortable your delivery will be, and the easier it will be for the baby to descend and be born. On the other hand, if you're keeping tension in your arm, your heart is probably tense and drawing up as well. As the muscles draw up and keep your baby in, the fall of your baby would be more difficult.

The more you practice, the more successful this exercise will be, much like arm stroking. The more your body recognizes that when your birth partner takes your wrist to lift your arm, you are to hand over the weight of your arm to your birth partner and let go of any stress, the faster your body can react. It has the ability to function effectively at the right time and, like arm stroking, can be used as a standalone relaxation trigger as well as within the framework of the relaxation script.

Many aspects of our actions are influenced in ways we aren't even aware of. We are very sensitive to patterns and routine as humans, so try to integrate your relaxation practice into your everyday routine, and it will become second nature. You might, for example, set aside some time each evening before going to bed to practice relaxation. Before bed is a great time to practice because you should be nice and comfortable and ready to sleep by the time you've completed the exercises. The activity also has immediate benefits, so it shouldn't feel like a chore; instead, make it something you look forward to doing each evening because it's fun and feels good, and it'll soon become as automatic as brushing your teeth.

If you take a moment to think about it, you can possibly think of a few things you already do in your life that cause you to respond in a certain way. These stimuli could be noises or smells; they could wake us up or put us to sleep; they could make us happy or sad; they could make us feel energized or hungry. You are using it as part of your birth planning if you have a daily relaxing activity at home. Since you've been doing it for years, it'll be efficient. If an existing organization exists, there is no need to create a new one. All you have to do now is figure out how to incorporate what you already do at home to ease into your birth.

Always keep in mind that the ultimate objective is to be relaxed both mentally and physically. It's less important how you get there. It's more important that you get there! Try some of the ideas in this book, as well as some of the stuff you already do, and you'll find that you have a toolbox full of things you can use in the field.

MASSAGE WITH LIGHT PRESSURE

The term "massage" is a little misleading since this method is more about light touch than conventional massage. This isn't a deep-tissue massage, and the thumbs aren't pressed into the muscle.

Instead, your birth partner will lightly brush your back with the backs of their hands, trailing their fingers slowly and lightly against your skin.

So, birth partners always begin at the base of the spine, just above the coccyx, with both hands. Then, as if drawing the lower layers of a palm tree's leaves, you shift your hands up the spine, the backs of your fingertips in light contact with the skin, before branching out. Start at the bottom and work your way up a little more, branching out and letting the backs of your fingertips trail down Mum's side gently. Start at the bottom and work your way up a little higher before branching out, around, and down. Until branching out over the tops of Mum's shoulders, continue until you hit the base of her spine (see the illustration overleaf). Then, starting at the bottom, go through the exercise again and again. Maintain a gentle touch and step slowly and softly. As you go, imagine drawing a palm tree on Mum's back.

It may seem monotonous or as though you aren't doing anything at all, but ideally, Mum can experience a pleasant tingling sensation distributed across her body – this is oxytocin. You can stimulate the synthesis of oxytocin and endorphins by stimulating the nerve endings in the spine. Endorphins are the body's own painkillers, and they're thought to be hundreds of times more powerful than morphine. Endorphins stay in the body for a long time and make you feel healthy, so the more of them you get, the better.

Light-touch massage is close to how a TENS machine works (Transcutaneous Electrical Nerve Stimulation). A TENS machine consists of four sticky pads that are mounted on your lower back and are connected to a small, handheld device by wires. You can then regulate the frequency of the rhythmic electrical pulse by turning it up or down. When you experience a surge, you can click the boost button on the unit. The rhythm changes as you push the boost button, and a new feeling spreads across your back. It takes some getting used to at first, but after a while, you'll almost forget about it. In terms of pain relief, the electric pulse causes the nerves to produce endorphins in the same way as light-touch massage does. A TENS machine designed specifically for labour and delivery can be purchased in pharmacies or rented from a variety of locations. Your midwife should be able to provide you with some guidance. You want one that is safe to use during pregnancy because there are other forms available for people with back pain that function in the same way but aren't safe to use during pregnancy.

My personal favorite is light-touch massage, which birth partners should do in between spikes to help Mum relax and develop more of the healthy, happy hormones. The TENS system can also help with this, and it can be used at home in both early and later stages of labour. The only position a TENS computer cannot be used is in a birth tub, for obvious reasons! Other advantages of the TENS machine include the fact that nothing is passed to the infant, unlike a drug, and that if you don't like it, you can easily turn it off rather than waiting for it to leave your system. It's entirely up to you if you want to use light-touch massage, a TENS unit, or a combination of both.

You should be starting to feel like you're putting together a decent toolkit for giving birth by now. Give each exercise a fair shot, even though it seems silly or counterproductive at first. It's possible that you're learning new things that you've never done before, so it'll take some time to get used to them or warm up to them. However, if you've tried something a few times and it's still not helping you relax, you can abandon it and concentrate on the strategies that do. It's fine as long as you have a few resources to focus on to help you relax. Never lose sight of the game's main goal: to unwind. It makes no difference how you get there. You may or may not use an arm drop. You might try something completely different. You may personalize your toolkit by using relaxation methods that you already use. It doesn't matter how you get there; what matters is that you get there. I hope that at least some of these methods assist you in achieving that wonderful state of relaxation. Breathing exercises, as well as counting or visualizations, are essential to learning and should be used during each surge. Between surges, you can use light-touch massage, guided relaxations, arm-stroking, and arm-drop techniques to help you deepen your relaxation and let go of any stress you picked up during the surge.

USING COMMON SENSE

We've already established how crucial it is to be at ease during childbirth. In a nutshell, the more relaxed you are, the higher your oxytocin levels would be. This hormone not only helps to speed up labour and make birth easier, but it also helps to minimize blood loss after birth, supports breastfeeding, and decreases the risk of postnatal depression. It also feels nice to be comfortable (bonus), and being relaxed in your body on a muscular level allows everything to soften, open, and release as it should.

When you're nervous or afraid, your body produces adrenaline and goes into fight or flight mode, which means your blood (carrying all that lovely and much-needed oxygen) is diverted away from the uterus muscles and toward your arms and legs. The uterus muscles become less powerful and painful as a result, and development slows – or even stops (not so good). With less blood and oxygen to the uterus, the baby is more likely to be distressed, which causes the mother-to-be to panic even more, causing more adrenaline to be released and the mother-to-be to join the awful cycle of terror tension, and pain.

As a result, we should all accept that the aim of the labour game is to stay as calm as possible. We've already discussed how relaxation techniques can improve, but there's another easy thing you can do: change your surroundings.

If it's the best option for you, staying at home is ideal: it's already a (hopefully) calming and familiar atmosphere. However, home may not be a choice or a place where you feel comfortable or secure for a variety of reasons. But it's not just doom and gloom – far from it! The good news is that you can do a lot to make your birthing space feel relaxed, comfortable, and familiar, regardless of where you choose to give birth (theatre included).

You can use the word "secure" a lot in your writing. The explanation for this is that when we feel safe, we are more likely to relax. When we feel challenged, though, we are unlikely to be able to relax. As a result, deciding when to give birth and maintaining a healthy environment is crucial.

When it comes to giving birth, feeling uninhibited is also vital because it allows you to relax and go with the flow completely. As a result, think about how the atmosphere (and the people in it) affects how you feel: you'll feel more self-conscious and inhibited if you're aware you're being watched (especially by strangers) and feel under observation or strain, or if you're in a brightly lit room. This is why it's crucial to think about how you want your birthing room to look and who you want to be there!

So, how do you make even the most clinical of environments feel secure, calm, and comfortable?

Everything boils down to our senses! We use our five senses to 'read' our surroundings or the space around us: sight, smell, sound, taste, and touch. We sometimes ingest all of this knowledge without realizing it, but it shapes how we feel in any given room, at any given time.

We simply need to ensure that each of our five senses is met with something that gives us comfort and helps us relax in order to turn a space into an oasis of peace and tranquility.

Since our senses are always heightened during labour, anything you do to promote relaxation and comfort will be amplified.

I want you to consider what you would like to see, hear, smell, taste, and touch that would make you feel calm, comfortable, and relaxed, using the five senses as a guide.

SIGHT

What would you like to see in the space? What would you like to see that would make you feel more at ease? Low lighting is preferred by the majority of people. It is well understood that dimming the lights makes you feel more relaxed and less inhibited or self-conscious. The good news is that dimmable lighting is available in most birth centers (and even some labour wards). In any case, having a small box of battery-operated tea lights to ensure you have a way to regulate the lighting is a good idea. When turned on in a dark room, they appear to be very realistic (despite being plastic). Since you can't have an open flame in a hospital or birth center, I prefer battery-operated ones over actual ones. And if you're planning a home birth, having them on hand as a backup is a smart idea in case you need to transfer in or your candles burn out.

Fairy lights are another choice, but the benefit of battery-operated tea lights is that they don't need an electrical outlet to run, and most people equate candlelight with romantic, intimate occasions – when they're relaxed and producing oxytocin, of course!

Other items you would like to see include familiar objects, such as pictures of your older children if you have them, or positive affirmation cards that you can scatter around the space.

It doesn't matter what it is as long as it makes you feel happy and calm.

SMELL

The smell is extremely evocative, and even the tiniest whiff of a scent can evoke long-forgotten memories. It's a powerful piece of work.

When it comes to birth, we want to harness this power and use it to offer relaxation and comfort, as we've said many times before. You don't want to smell like a hospital or cleaning products – or something less savory for that matter!

Essential oils are wonderful, particularly lavender and chamomile, which are known to help with relaxation. (However, be aware that certain essential oils are not approved for use during pregnancy, so double-check before using them.)

If you're at home, you can always buy an essential oil room spray or place them in a diffuser or oil burner. Alternatively, you can already have a favorite scented candle that you use to unwind. Rollerballs, which you can use to add essential oils to your pulse points like perfume securely, are perfect because they are very compact, as are room sprays.

Many essential oil-based room sprays have a luxurious spa scent. Even if they haven't had many spa vacations, most people will equate the spa-like scent with relaxation and optimistic, pleasant thoughts, so something like this would be ideal.

Whatever you decide, make sure you have a way to make the room smell good by using a perfume that brings back happy memories of relaxing times. Giving a room a fast spritz is a simple and quick way to change the atmosphere. It will help you sleep better if you close your eyes and breathe deeply.

SOUND

When you're in labour, what do you want to hear? Do you want to hear about people's weekend plans or what they plan to do after work? Do you want to be mindful of what's going on in the world around you? Conversations with other women and healthcare providers? Most likely not. Remember, what would make you relax more deeply?

Since music can be played by many people, creating a playlist with a combination of cheerful, positive tunes and calmer, calming music is a good idea. Favorite songs are also associated with happier memories, so include them. Music, like a smell, has the ability to take you to a different place and time. Make sure the location and time are appropriate!

Others would enjoy listening to guided relaxations or positive affirmations, particularly if they have already done so while pregnant. The audio will be very familiar to you, and hearing it during labour will be reassuring.

Others will choose to play generic background music, such as spa music. You might almost imagine you were on a spa break with your eyes closed and the combination of gentle pan-pipe music and the scent of essential oils filling the room! Any of these items can seem insignificant on their own, but when taken together, they can make a significant difference in how comfortable you feel.

When you're in labour, you should listen to any of the above, alternating between your favorite songs, optimistic affirmations, directed relaxations, and spa music. Simply make sure the tracks are ready to play on your phone or another computer, and pack either a small portable speaker or a pair of headphones (or both) in your birth bag so you can listen on the big day.

TASTE

What would you eat to make you feel better and more content? When it comes to the big day, what are you most excited to open? Remember that labour is similar to a workout in that your uterus muscles will be working hard for a long time, so eat plenty of calories and stay hydrated. Would you run a marathon on an empty stomach?

So bring plenty of beverages – water, coconut water, maybe a can of something fizzy – as well as non-perishable snacks for when you're in labour. Make sure you pack a treat for yourself – if there was ever a time for a little reward, now is it!

TIP: While we're on the subject of food and drink, make sure your birth partner has enough supplies for himself or herself. Nothing is more aggravating than a grumpy birth partner!

TOUCH

What would you put on that will make you feel good? Consider fabrics that are either cool or warm, depending on the season. Consider the clothes you normally put on when you want to unwind. If you're going to use a birth pool, think about what you'll wear – maybe a bikini top?

Remember that the most important thing is that you feel at ease, relaxed, unrestricted, and not self-conscious. If at all possible, avoid wearing a hospital gown, as this would send the message to your mind that you are a patient and that something is wrong, as these are the common associations we have with hospital gowns, and they are deeply ingrained in our subconscious. If you are admitted to the hospital, you can be given one, but you can still opt to wear your own clothing.

A dressing gown and slippers, a simple oversized cotton T-shirt, baggy tracksuit bottoms, your PJs, or even a summer dress might be appropriate. It is completely up to you to make your decision.

You may also want to bring a pillow or a blanket or something else that makes you feel more relaxed and comfortable. Familiar objects are particularly beneficial because you already have a lot of positive experiences with them.

Don't forget about the massage oil. This will come under the category of contact. Many massage oils have essential oils that are safe to use during pregnancy and can help you relax. You could use one of those, or you could use a tub of pure coconut oil. Coconut oil is excellent for massage and is extremely moisturizing for the skin, as well as conjuring up images of pia Coladas due to its scent! Anything that reminds us of summer vacation drinks (or mocktails) is usually a positive thing.

That's what there is to it. Sight, Sound, Smell, Taste, and Touch: the five senses and a simple checklist to ensure you're making a good impression.

A birth-friendly environment is one that feels relaxed and comfortable and allows you to let go and relax completely.

The beauty of this checklist is that it makes transforming a room so easy. And, best of all, it can be used anywhere: at home, in a birth center, or on a labour and delivery ward. You can change the entire atmosphere of a room in a matter of minutes, no matter where you are, as long as you have the bits and pieces in your birth bag. Switch on the lights, light your candles, spritz your room with room spray, put on your comfiest, and soak it all in a while, sipping coconut water and munching on jelly babies! Even the most clinical of spaces can be turned into a romantic and intimate spa setting.

CHAPTER EIGHT

TURNING A BIRTH PARTNER INTO A HYPNOBIRTH PARTNER

Your position as a birth companion is extremely critical. You'll be your partner's emotional and physical support when she gives birth to the infant. You may have read or attended antenatal classes to prepare, or you may feel unprepared. The emphasis of mindful hypnobirthing planning is on emotional preparation and learning to be a strong and centered spouse, free of your own judgment and concerns about birth.

WHAT KIND OF BIRTH PARTNER DO YOU CHOOSE?

Women used to give birth near their mothers, sisters, and aunts until the last century. People have migrated to cities where jobs are located away from their traditional family units as the economy has grown and become more industrialized. In today's world, this means that a birth partner is more likely to become a life partner. It is important for a woman to feel safe and secure while giving birth. According to research, a trusted female, in keeping with tradition, independent of the family, gives reliably better birth results, but a well-prepared birth partner may be just as successful in the absence of this.

Both parents are present at their baby's birth and hold them shortly after having feelings of bonding that are very close to those experienced by mothers during the first two weeks. This event has been shown to have a long-term impact, with parents who were present at birth becoming more interested in their children as they grow up. A parent who is actively involved, emotionally committed, and connected in their children's lives will only support the child and the family unit.

The value of a successful birth partner is immeasurable. You can be the best possible help if you are both relaxed, know what your job is, and can let go of the need to manage the space based on your own needs. You will be the vehicle that helps carry her and your baby on their birth journey if you fully trust your wife and care for her during her baby's birth with loving-kindness, compassion, and determination.

PARTNERS HAVE CHOICES TOO

People always talk about mothers exercising their rights and being in charge of their children's births, but we seldom hear about their partners' wishes. It will affect the birth if you do not want to be present at the birth or if some aspects of the birth make you unhappy. You'll almost certainly release adrenaline, which can be felt by those in the room and has the potential to influence how the mother feels and how her body reacts to birth. If you don't want to see your baby's birth in every detail – which is not uncommon – you should be respected. This, too, should be valued if you don't want to cut the cord. While some overzealous midwives demand that the father be present when the baby is born, and unwilling partners are pulled down to cut the cord.

YOUR REQUIREMENTS MUST ALSO BE MET

Don't take it personally if your partner doesn't want you there for some reason. Have a conversation about it. Some women are unable to let go completely in front of their partner or someone else. Talking about why you're doing it and being honest about how you both feel will help you get stronger.

EMOTIONAL PREPARATION

Spending time dwelling on your baby and your partner's pregnancy will help you emotionally prepare. Take some time together to learn about your kid, as well as to talk to your baby. While any parent will do this naturally, they will read the football score to their child, sing to them, or play music for them. Although a baby does not hear sounds in the same way as we do, they are aware of subtle variations in cadence, or language rhythm, that are special to each person. Certain rhythms are calming to babies; studies show that babies are very aware of rhythm and can remember specific pieces of music, ranging from soap opera theme tunes to baroque, so the rhythm of the parent's voice is very familiar and comforting to them. Babies turn or shift their heads in the direction of the voice. Even after they are born, a baby who has heard their parent talk directly to the belly button on a regular basis may know their voice and feel calmer when it is near them.

Making the bond with your baby on a regular basis and accepting them as a member of your family while they are still in the womb can help you gradually adapt to having another person in your relationship. Make sure you spend time with your wife doing some of the activities in this book so you can form a bond with her and the baby and learn how to assist her in these techniques.

Appointments for antenatal care should be scheduled ahead of time.

Discuss your partner's antenatal appointments with her and schedule some time off to accompany her to these appointments, even though they are routine. In the UK, you have the legal right to take time off for antenatal appointments, but your employer is not required to pay you for this time off; some employers do or simply allow you to make up the time. Being able to regularly listen to your baby's heartbeat and being a part of those appointments can be an easy but powerful way to bond emotionally with your baby.

In one character, you can play three different roles.

You may have an idea of what to expect at birth if you've taken NHS or NCT courses. Whether you're doing hypnobirthing or mindfully planning, your method would be slightly different. The birthing partner has three responsibilities:

- The Practical Partner
- The Protective Partner
- The Mindful Partner

These three tasks specifically describe the various facets of a birthing partner's work, all of which help mum relax and trust that everything will be taken care of. Every couple's details for these three jobs will be different, so it's up to you to sit down and go through the details that are important to you.

THE PRACTICAL PARTNER

This position is all about practical work, as you might have guessed. When your wife is going through the birth process, it's important that you don't ask her where everything is or how things should be. Some practical tasks, such as ensuring that the bag is in the car and that you have enough money for parking, are self-evident. Others, such as setting up the room according to what you've learned in this book, might require a little more thought. Massage and physical contact are examples of more hands-on activities included in the practical aspect.

THE PRACTICAL PARTNER CHECKLIST

- Lights off in the room
- Aromatherapy oil
- Blanket/bedroom pillow
- Hypnosis tracks on CD and MP3 player, headphones
- Affirmations
- Money

THE PROTECTIVE PARTNER

The majority of people believe that this is the most difficult position. When a woman enters the facility, she may be required to walk through four or five gates that belong to someone else. There's the hospital entrance, reception, doors to the birthing suite, possibly another set of doors to the midwifery- or consultancy-led unit, and finally, the room itself. The midwife was well aware that the mother would be in an unfamiliar environment. It is her right to have someone serve as her gatekeeper so that she feels protected and that someone she can trust is watching out for her.

When your partner is in her birthing zone, it's also vital to be the gatekeeper. Slowing down neo-cortical behavior is the aim in order to hold her in that condition. Questions from medical personnel and interactions with her mother all cause her neo-cortex, causing her inner narrator to come to life. It can jolt her out of her birthing zone if the room is dark and someone turns on a light; or if many people rush into the room, it can imbue a feeling of being observed, triggering her alarm systems and 'waking' her up.

The gatekeeper's role is to ensure that the birth wishes are followed. If your birth wishes to state, "Could you talk to my partner before interrupting me?" the staff should first speak with you. They cannot give her pain relief if her birth preferences state, "Please do not offer me pain relief; I will ask for it if I need it," and it is your responsibility to ensure that this is followed.

COMMUNICATION IS ESSENTIAL

Before the mother has to be contacted, a birthing partner may be able to speak with the midwives or doctors and buy time or refuse an intervention depending on the birth wishes and conversations the couple had prior to the birth. Allowing themselves to think, "I'm not a doctor or a midwife, I don't have medical training, how do I make these choices?" is a challenge for many people. It may be complicated, but you do not need to be a medical professional to make decisions; all you need is enough information about the benefits and risks to make an informed decision.

We spoke about the BRAINS issues. This is a very well-specified collection of questions that allows you to get the details you need to make a decision and is given out in several antenatal classes around the world. The question to ask if the birth has slowed and they want to speed it up is, "Is mum fine, and is the baby fine?" If you answered yes, consider why that intervention is needed. Always keep in mind that the philosophy of natural birth is birth without interruption. Yes, birth can take a long time and be unpredictably unpredictable, so patience is essential. If all is well, consider why you need this intervention. You may be told that there are many things that may go wrong, particularly if the medical team is recommending you to have a specific operation, but remember that everything is fine right now. This will allow you to pass the time while keeping the mother's space free of anxiety or concern. You should be assured that if anything goes wrong, the medical staff can respond quickly.

The gatekeeper's other responsibility is to establish a rapport with your midwife. It's not unusual for midwives to feel uneasy when they're speaking on behalf of their partner: they're used to talking to the mother and are prepared to develop rapport with her. This is where unspoken contact will become problematic. It can be unsettling if the midwife is busy, dismissive, or not really listening to the couple's wishes. It takes experience and empathy to be able to turn off from one couple to really be with another couple a few minutes later in a crowded hospital unit where she might be caring for multiple couples. The instinct of a birthing partner to protect his partner is powerful. When this occurs, our body language changes; we can release adrenaline and become more aggressive; as a result, the midwife may become anxious and perceive the couple as demanding and uncooperative.

BEING AN EMPATHETIC COMMUNICATOR

Engaging with the midwife compassionately, perhaps asking for her advice and expertise in helping you remain as true to your birth preferences as possible, will make all the difference.

Make sure your body language says, "I am open to your ideas, and I am interested in hearing what you have to say." Tilt your head to one side, which subconsciously signals to her that you are paying attention to her. If she says she's busy, use reflective language like this: 'I understand you're busy; when you're ready...' Midwives aren't invincible, even though they seem to be at times; they're human beings under stress who react to recognition and empathy. She could be newly educated and afraid of doing something she hasn't done before; she could be sick, or she could be distracted by an emergency in another room.

This is one of the most important days of your life. Your child is about to be born; don't you think you deserve complete attention and that the midwife should be there for you when you need her?

The reality is that hospitals are understaffed, and midwives are under pressure at work, which has an effect on how well they will care for you. There is likely to be less pressure to consider interference if you have a home birth, and one-on-one treatment makes it much easier to form a bond with your midwife, who might be more relaxed and at ease in your home.

THE PROTECTIVE PARTNER CHECKLIST

- ☐ ☐ BRAINS
- ☐ ☐ Practice the exercise 'Three, two, one, relax, relax, relax.'
- ☐ ☐ Three copies of your birth preferences
- ☐ ☐ Any research that supports choices important to you**The Conscious Partner**

All of your realistic and constructive assistance is critical in ensuring that the climate is perfect. This helps your partner to relax and let go of any worries or anxieties completely. It's possible that your wife won't want to speak or converse when she's giving birth. She'll be in her birthing zone if she's using hypnobirthing. You might notice when she's having a contraction, or you might not.

Being in the birthing zone doesn't mean she'll be absolutely still or that she won't ask you questions or talk to you. Some women may converse in between contractions, while others may tend to ask questions without anticipating a response. A partner's natural instinct is to respond to those questions directly.

BIRTH TALK, SLEEP TALK

When women are in the throes of labour, it's common for them to speak in a sleepy manner. Rather than asking her what she wants or offering suggestions, simply take her head in your hands, smile, and tell her if she can do it, 'You think you can't do this, but you can.' I'm with you; you're a smart woman. A simple constructive suggestion that does not involve an answer will usually suffice. And nonverbal responses have a lot of control. Looking into your partner's eyes, holding her hands, and smiling reassuringly after each contraction or when she opened her eyes would send a very powerful message that everything is fine, you're doing well, I love you, and I'm here for you.

PRESENCE

All it takes is a solid, quiet presence to make a difference. Birth may be fast or slow, but knowing that someone is watching out for you and checking for danger can lower the mother's adrenaline and nor-adrenaline levels, enabling labour to progress. This may include just sitting quietly and being present at the moment, whether awake or asleep in the chair next to her.

You will train yourself to be a mindful partner by using any of the hypnosis methods in this book. You may also try the exercise below. You may also bring something with you, such as a book, crossword puzzles, or Sudoku puzzles. Be mindful, however, that partners using phones or computers when giving birth have had a negative reaction!

I'M TERRIFIED OF SEEING MY PARTNER HURT

A partner's natural instinct is to protect and care about the person they love. For others, the most difficult part is seeing someone they care about go through such physical pain and not knowing how to help. A birth partner's natural instinct may be to want to be the "rescuer." Seeing the person they care for behaving out of character will make them feel uneasy. One of the most common issues among partners who attend my classes is this.

Birth is a life-changing event. Your wife may not be in pain, even though your impression is that she is. The reactions of a partner are founded on preconceptions and beliefs about birth based on what they've heard secondhand or seen on TV.

What would you see if you were lucky enough to witness a woman give birth unassisted in a location she chose? You'll be taken aback by her intensity at first. As she sits, sways, and squats to find the best place to ease her baby out, her thighs stand firm and mighty like those of a fighter. Then you'll hear her make deep primal noises as she works, sounds that come from her abdomen rather than her throat as she grunts and moans with exertion: sounds that are rarely heard except in the most uninhibited of love-making. Maybe you won't note the glistening river of mucus tinged with blood and the waters that flow down her thighs unnoticed: she's stepped into another plane of life and is beyond seeing those things. Finally, her beauty will strike you: her face softened by the rush of oxytocin, her eyes wide and sparkling, her pupils dark, deep, and open. And you'll think to yourself – how could you not? – what a magnificent creature a woman is. But you'll only be able to see this incredible sight if you realize that if you interfere with her job, she'll be thrown off track.

WHAT DO I DO IF I GET ANXIOUS?

You do not know how to cope with your partner's natural need to make noise and show herself in a more extroverted manner. Your first reaction could be to give pain medication, even though she has said that she does not want it, or to believe that something is wrong and become concerned. The presumption that something is wrong will cause the birth partner to release adrenaline, which the mother can pick up on an unconscious level.

If this happens, it's important that you're able to recognize the emotion that's emerging inside you and give your partner the room she needs to express herself in the way she wants to: without judgment.

Her contractions can become stronger and longer as the birth progresses. They may appear to be getting closer; at times, it may even appear as though they are colliding. Even if she has been coping well up to this stage, your wife can suggest she can no longer do it. She will demand an epidural and be adamant about getting one. It's very likely that you're in the transition stage. Since there is a normal rush of adrenaline at a particular point during birth, midwives can easily detect a woman in transition. Even women who have been breathing in a very concentrated manner can unexpectedly shift.

This can be difficult for the birth partner, but it's important that your partner uses some of the strategies you learned when planning for a hypnobirthing at this stage. Many of the strategies will help you be emotionally present for your partner. You can do this with your partner, who will benefit from your ability to remain focused, relaxed, and calm.

CHAPTER NINE

WHEN WILL BIRTH BEGIN?

Your body is quietly preparing for your baby's birth as you practice your hypnosis exercises every day, preparing your mind for birth. Many of these subtle changes in your body go unnoticed because hormones activate modifications that are perfectly tailored to your body and your infant. Knowing what your hormones are doing and being mindful of physical changes will help you direct and educate yourself on how things are changing in preparation for birth.

THE LAST WEEKS OF YOUR PREGNANCY

Every woman gives birth in her own 'uniquely natural' way, just like you. Being aware of the interconnectedness of your body's, baby's, and brain's hormonal balance will help you gain trust in whatever direction you want to give birth. Each woman's sensitivity to her own hormones is special, and her hormonal balance is ideal for her.

YOUR HORMONES ARE CHANGING

As you go about your everyday routine, your hormones are busy preparing your body for conception, pregnancy, and birth. You'd be surprised if you knew how busy your body was! It's like being in a big train station, with hormones on the move, traveling to various locations in preparation for the birth of your infant. Their travels, arrivals, and departures are all scheduled around specific times. The trains are sometimes late; maybe they are on a slow cross-country line. Consider your brain planning and organizing all of those various journeys; it's a difficult job, but it gets the job done. Allowing it to run its course is the best option. It's critical to understand your hormones, and it's particularly important to do so about 37 weeks pregnant.

You are the hormones, and their exchange is so special, precise, and delicate that it is difficult to modify or correctly interfere with it. Consider a clock with a complex movement, and each part is programmed to keep the others in place so that the whole works in unison to bring you the perfect time. Understanding how hormonal shifts cause familiar changes during pregnancy will really help you see how capable your body is of beginning birth and doing it in the most relaxed and safe way for you and your infant.

WHAT HAPPENS TO THE HORMONES DURING PREGNANCY AND AFTER BIRTH?

Relaxin, which is formed by the corpus luteum, breasts, and placenta, is released in the weeks leading up to your baby's birth. Relaxin levels peak around 14 weeks of pregnancy, right around the time your baby is due to arrive. Heartburn and pelvic pain are two symptoms of relaxin. Relaxin softens the ligaments in your pelvis, allowing more room for the baby to move through the vaginal opening. Relaxin also softens the cervix in preparation for birth, which may happen a few weeks before the due date. Relaxin may also be the hormone responsible for vasodilation, which helps dilate blood vessels and lower blood pressure, according to new studies. This is important because your blood volume rises by 40–50% during pregnancy to handle changes in your body and control nutrition for your infant.

Progesterone is a hormone that rises during pregnancy to help soften muscles in the womb so that the baby can develop. It also protects the placenta by fending off unwanted cells and enhances the mucosal lining, which is part of the mucus plug and helps prevent infection from entering the womb.

Before birth, progesterone levels begin to drop, signaling estrogen to rise. Progesterone and estrogen act in tandem. Progesterone is a crucial hormone during conception and pregnancy since it aids in the growth of the womb lining and prevents menstruation. It also aids in the baby's nutrition and acts in tandem with estrogen to prepare for breastfeeding.

Early in pregnancy, high levels of the hormone hCG help ensure that the corpus luteum continues to release high levels of progesterone until the placenta takes over progesterone development. The corpus luteum is a mini hormone exchange in your ovary that temporarily helps and maintains a pregnancy-friendly atmosphere before the placenta develops and takes over. Common pregnancy symptoms include nausea, headaches, food cravings, tiredness, and breast tenderness as a result of these hormone changes. When progesterone is released from the placenta, hCG levels begin to drop in the third and fourth months, and symptoms begin to fade.

OESTROGEN

Oestrogen is a crucial hormone during pregnancy since it promotes the development of the uterus, breasts, and breast ducts, all of which aid in the production of milk and prepare you for breastfeeding. It also raises the number of oxytocin receptors and 'gap junctions' in your womb lining and around your cervix, which increases contraction power. These gap junctions are extremely important; they serve as contact hubs during your baby's birth, acting as a telephone exchange between all of the various hormones and aiding in the regulation of contractions as well as the softening and opening of your cervix.

YOUR HORMONES WHEN YOU GET READY TO HAVE A BABY

Both estrogen and progesterone levels rise during pregnancy, but progesterone levels start to fall after the seventh month, while estrogen levels continue to rise. This is in preparation for birth, as a higher estrogen ratio allows your womb to soften, expand, and contract more effectively. It's amazing how the body's hormones reverse their work thanks to the contact centers set up during pregnancy. Hormones that helped keep your cervix closed and your baby healthy during their nine months in your womb start to decline, whereas those that help soften your body tissues in preparation for birth increase.

As progesterone levels drop, the increasing estrogen released by the placenta triggers the release of prostaglandins, which encourages birth to begin. Prostaglandins are messengers found in the tissues surrounding your cervix that help push the start button for birth by relaying signals between your cervix, womb, and brain. If you are past your due date, your midwife will give you a sweep. She will try to start your contractions by sweeping her fingertips around your cervix and an amniotic sack. If you have opted to have a sweep, you are most likely very close to giving birth, and these hormonal exchanges would have already begun days, if not weeks before you give birth. When the midwife tells you that your cervix is soft and small, it means that your body's hormones have already begun to prepare for birth.

During pregnancy, the mucus plug is a jelly-like material that serves as a barrier and is kept in place by your cervix, which is closed. The loss of some of your mucus plug, also known as your 'show,' is another indication that your hormones are preparing your body for the birth of your infant. The plug loosens, and pieces of it will slip away as your cervix softens and thins. You may or may not see it; it may be as simple as a thick, clear vaginal discharge, or it may be thick and streaked with blood. This is natural and can occur weeks, days, or hours before birth, but it often indicates that your body's hormones are preparing you and your baby for birth.

Imagine your fist is closed tight, like your cervix, and you have some egg white in it, then slowly and gently open your fist. Some of the egg white will slip away when your fist opens entirely, but not all of it.

WHAT CAUSES LABOUR TO BEGIN?

Labour is triggered by a complex exchange of hormones between your baby and your body, and it is timed specifically for you and your baby. Until recently, it was assumed that the baby was the catalyst for this sequence of events. However, evidence suggests that labour may be caused when your baby's energy demands begin to exceed what your body can support.

Only then will your baby prepare for birth by and androgen levels and releasing cortisol, both of which help your baby's lungs develop and prepare for life outside the womb.

When your baby's lungs receive this boost, it triggers hormonal changes in you, which trigger labour. A rise in prostaglandins can be noticeable because it often causes loose stools or diarrhea, which is a common indication that labour is about to begin. The region around your uterus and bowels is softening, opening, and relaxing in preparation for the birth of your infant. You may be shocked to learn that less than 60% of women perceive contractions as the beginning of their labour, instead of recognizing water breaking, loose stools, blood staining, emotional changes, or sleep disturbances as signs that labour has begun.

Prostaglandins, unlike other hormones, are messengers found in tissue all over the body and are not produced in the brain. They gather in large numbers around the cervix's tissue, preparing the cervix to open. The stretching and pressure from your baby's head cause the oxytocin receptors to spring into action and induce the release of oxytocin when the cervix expands and softens.

Contractions are triggered by the release of oxytocin, which causes more oxytocin to be released, resulting in more contractions. This is what is known as a positive feedback loop. Early labour contractions can be felt more in the lower part of your uterus as your cervix softens and thins in response to prostaglandins and low oxytocin levels. They are a sign that your body is getting its act together and beginning to stretch and expand, organizing its needs for labour. They are often referred to as tweaks and niggles by women and are a good sign that your body is getting its act together and starting to stretch and expand, coordinating its needs for labour. When labour progresses, oxytocin levels increase, and contractions get closer together. A pressure or tightening can now be felt more over the top half of your uterus, known as the fundal region.

IS THERE ANYTHING I CAN DO TO HELP MY BODY?

The first step is to pay attention to your body. Recognize these changes and shifts in your body as signs that you're approaching labour; each small change is a step along the road to your birth. Allow yourself to take in the scenery. Slow down; don't rush to get to your destination; allow your body to carry you along like your legs will on a stroll or a run. Have faith that you will arrive at your destination.

TAKE CARE OF YOUR BODY

Take care of your body as you would a child. Healthy eating will assist the body in achieving the best possible condition for birth. Some complications, such as pre-eclampsia – a severe complication that affects both the mother and the infant – have been linked to diet in studies. When you're in a good mood, you'll find that you instinctively gravitate toward healthy foods. When nervous or worried, some women don't eat properly; they either don't eat enough or eat too many of the wrong stuff, comfort foods. Make sure your diet is balanced and full of vegetables. Pay attention to what the body wants to consume and what it doesn't.

If you work out, don't stop just because you're pregnant; keep doing what you're doing. Keeping fit and safe is important, and it will also benefit you after your baby is born. Prenatal yoga and Pilates classes are becoming more common as a way to prepare for childbirth.

TAKE CARE OF YOUR MIND.

Even if you've struggled to fit it in before, at about 37 weeks, you can increase your mindful hypnobirthing practice and be doing it every day. To help you remember, use the Practice Guidelines on pages (43–4). Consider taking a break from work earlier. You may believe that working until the last minute buys you time later, but the weeks leading up to your baby's birth are crucial because they enable you to change and adapt to a slower pace of life. Even without the hormonal swings, stopping a busy career, going into labour, and caring for a baby in the span of a few days can be an emotional roller-coaster! Treat yourself and your hormones with respect. Relax and focus yourself before childbirth starts, and you become a mother to find a balance before your baby is born and enjoy the last few quiet weeks of pregnancy.

TAKING CARE OF THE NEW MOTHER

At this time, mindfulness will help you lean into your physical and emotional feelings. Keep an open mind about your emotions and consider them as a sign that you're in the midst of transitioning from pregnancy to motherhood. This period has also been given a name: 'Zwischen,' which means 'between' in German. It's a liminal period between pregnancy and birth, a period when you may feel as though you're caught in the middle of being a parent and not being a parent, of crossing the threshold from maidenhood to motherhood. Your body is softening and shifting, but it also appears that the souls of mother and child, both individually and as a family, are beginning to emerge from the womb. You can interact with this in-between period in a different way if you go deeper into yourself at this stage. Avoid worrying about when your baby will arrive during the time when your baby is due. Change the focus from what isn't happening to what is.

You will nurture your inner mother by taking care of her until you have a child to look after. Spend time doing activities that help you relax and unwind. It could be a long walk, a bath, or a massage. Make a list of stuff that would usually sound indulgent but that you can see as a way to show compassion and affection to the mother you'll be.

If you're on maternity leave, now is a great time to start planning for the postpartum era, thinking about how you can apply what you've learned in this book to parenthood. You can learn more about postnatal preparation by visiting.

THE WOBBLE OF 40 WEEKS

As the due date approaches, you will begin to feel nervous or anxious. And for people who have used hypnobirthing to plan, the '40-week wobble' pops up time and time again. It can happen at any point after 37 weeks. This is for a variety of reasons! To begin with, major changes are occurring; your brain is beginning to adjust in preparation for mothering your infant, allowing you to be alert and remember things like their cry. Your brain will be able to distinguish your baby's cry from a room full of other babies from the moment they are born. Isn't that amazing?

The second factor to be aware of is 'expectation anxiety,' which is extremely common in hypnotherapy, especially while dealing with fears that cannot be checked before the event occurs. Expectation anxiety is common for fear of flight, for example, because you don't know if the hypnotherapy methods will work until you're on the plane and in the air. Trust the process; once you've completed your training, everything will fall into place. Thousands of mothers have told me about their experiences.

It's important to keep your oxytocin levels up and your adrenaline levels down if you're experiencing this wobble. Remove as much stress as possible from this time. Remember your body's amazing ability to get it in the right place at the right time.

Consider the following oxytocin-inducing exercises:

- Go for a walk in the woods.
- Listen to the music on your MP3 player.
- Nipple stimulation (yes, it really works!) Reread the section on hormones.
- Feel free to add your own.

Baby will arrive at their own pace, so just surrender to it, let go of any fears, and let it happen.

CHAPTER TEN

THIS IS IT! SIGNS THAT LABOUR HAS STARTED

The signs that labour has begun may be perplexing. Labour doesn't start right away; it's a gradual series of changes and shifts in your body that you don't realize until you're convinced you're in labour. Physical shifts, such as your plug falling out, loose stools, niggles in your lower uterus, knowledge of the baby being very tiny, and maybe even a good night's sleep, are also signs of hormonal changes. Nature is generous in this way.

If your wife is a little disoriented and absent-minded than normal, it may be an indication that oxytocin levels are rising, and she is entering her birthing zone. Knowing when to call the midwife or go to the doctor, as well as recognizing the signs that the body is warming up, may be beneficial.

HOW WOULD I KNOW WHEN LABOUR HAS STARTED?

If you've already had a kid, you might be much more at ease when it comes to the start of labour. When one person's labour begins will be entirely different from when another begins.

One of the most common blunders made by first-time mothers is believing that they should go to the hospital as soon as anything happens. If you arrive at the hospital too early, labour may slow down temporarily as you become acquainted with the environment in which you will give birth, or it may be that labour hasn't yet found its rhythm and is simply warming up. This could lead to 'augmentation' or medical assistance to speed up or restart labour.

WARMING UP AND BRAXTON HICKS

Warm-up contractions are the name given to Braxton Hicks contractions since that is exactly what they are. Your body is getting ready to give birth. They may be a non-painful tightening, or you can need to concentrate on your breathing. They can begin weeks or days before the due date.

Braxton Hicks do not affect everybody, but they may sound like real contractions. They could be normal and last for a few hours before disappearing, only to reappear later that day or the next. If this happens to you, think of it as your body settling into a new routine. These contractions are similar to turning an engine over: it can take a few turns before the engine catches and starts.

Practice the techniques during these early warm-up contractions, pausing to pause in between. If they're really loud, take a shower or a bath. Go for a stroll or just carry on with your normal routine. Second-time mothers are often distracted by other items, particularly the treatment of other children, and miss these contractions, while a first-time mother is on the lookout for any sign, exaggerating what is really going on.

MY CHILD IS ENGAGING. SO, WHAT DOES THIS IMPLY?

Your midwife can tell you that your baby is active. This indicates that your baby is starting to descend into the pelvis in preparation for labour. This can happen weeks or days before the due date, or – particularly if you've already had children – right before the due date, sometimes even during labour. Your baby may engage in a way that makes you feel like he or she is about to fall out; some women claim they feel like their baby is about to fall out. They aren't going to! It may feel like you're having aches and pains and your baby is scrambling around, but note that if your baby is engaged, their head is fitted into your pelvis, and their movement is limited.

Braxton Hicks contractions may be mistaken for early labour by first-time mothers. You'll know you're in labour when the contractions get heavier and last longer. Some women's contractions maybe five minutes apart for the duration of their labour; others may begin at ten minutes apart, progress to seven minutes apart, and finally to three minutes apart. 'Is there three in ten or four in ten?' a midwife might ask, referring to whether there are three contractions in ten minutes or four contractions in ten minutes.

The niggles in your uterus start to form a clear pattern and migrate up into your abdomen. Through each contraction, your belly tightens, pressing your baby's head against your cervix. It's like giving your baby a big hug. Your cervix opens a little more each time your baby's head presses down on it.

This is why location is so critical, and early labour movement will definitely help jiggle babies around, so they get into the ideal position. When your baby is in a good spot, the head is snugly against the cervix, allowing the cervix to open gently and easily. You should start using the strategies as labour progress; however, if the contractions are spaced far apart, you will still be able to do other things. When the contractions are still far apart and last less than a minute, you can find that you can comfortably breathe through them and get on with your life. Remember what you know about concentration and how you can amplify something by focusing on it. As your labour progresses, you will find yourself focusing more and more on yourself.

When contractions begin, you might be able to cook some meals, do some laundry or ironing, or even go for a walk or go shopping while pausing to breathe through them.

Then, as they grow longer, bigger, or closer together, you may choose to remain in your home. This is also when women really nest, finishing up any last-minute preparations around the house. You could take a shower or a bath and listen to your hypnosis tracks when doing so.

You may feel as if the contractions are waves and that you are simply riding them as you remain centered and centered in your birthing region, using breathing, affirmations, and loving massage, as well as listening to your hypnosis tracks. You should be in sync with your body's rhythm when you enter your birthing region, allowing your contractions to pass through your body and carry your baby to you.

KEEPING TRACK OF YOUR CONTRACTIONS

Each contraction will last anywhere from 40 seconds to an hour and a half. And if you have three contractions every ten minutes, your body will have about six minutes to rest every ten minutes. Your body will contract for three hours and rest for seven hours if you were in labour for ten hours and contracting three minutes apart. The time between contractions is crucial when practicing conscientious hypnobirthing. Your muscles are able to let go between contractions if you are relaxed and floppy, rather than keeping on to stress. Between contractions, the tension in your body can cause excessive pain.

Your body should relax fully between contractions, regardless of how painful they are, if you are not tense. The jaw and facial muscles of a woman in labour who is relaxed between contractions would be very relaxed. This is significant because the tension in your jaw reflects the tension in your pelvic region. If you relax your neck, your pelvic region will relax as well.

PUTTING YOUR TRAINING TO WORK

Oxytocin levels would have started to increase by the time you go into labour, and your contractions start. Beta-endorphins will start to circulate, allowing your body to relax into the rhythm of your contractions and preparing you for labour.

Contractions are like waves; you can sense them coming on, so you have a few moments to compose yourself, center yourself, breathe deeply, and concentrate before they happen. You can feel tightness around your bump and a heavy squeezing as the contraction progresses. Your bump can simply harden in early labour, similar to a Braxton Hicks contraction. Your contraction builds up, peaks, and then fades away, just like a wave. Even if the contraction lasts a minute and a half, it only increases for half the time, peaking in seconds. As she felt her contraction fade away, one woman told me that her body relaxed and her leg muscles felt a profound sense of release.

WHICH CONTRACTIONS TECHNIQUES WORK BEST?

Focus on your breathing, your mantra, and your breathing in 'three, two, one' and breathing out 'relax, relax, relax' during contractions. Use your hypnosis deepener and ask your partner to count down for you if you need help staying focused in your birthing zone. They may place a strong hand on your back, which is comforting and soothing. Consider some of the anchors you've learned at this stage.

If you're experiencing back pain, have your partner apply pressure to your lower back, just above your buttocks. In your lower back, you can also use a massage roller ball to apply pressure where it's needed. Ask your midwife for assistance if your partner isn't sure what to do. Warmth in the lower back will provide a great deal of relief.

Movement is also beneficial. During contractions, you may feel compelled to shift, whether it's bending forward and swaying your hips from side to side, sitting on a ball and rocking your pelvis, or even stamping from one foot to the other, as some women do. Did you know that there are ancient belly dancing moves that can help move the baby down during labour?

IS IT NECESSARY FOR ME TO BE ON THE MOVE ALL OF THE TIME?

During labour, movement is extremely necessary because it aids in the positioning of the infant. Running or swaying makes the baby relax into the pelvis and wriggle down because of the normal rocking action. Walking meditation is a perfect way to remain healthy and in your birthing zone when you're in labour. The following mindful movement exercise is ideal for use during labour because it allows you to interact with the energy of contractions.

If you're exhausted or need a break, there's nothing wrong with lying down for a while. You can relax while still having contractions if you lie on your left side with your headphones on and listen to your hypnosis songs. It's much preferable to feel rested rather than tired and worried about needing to stay upright and going.

You are in the moment while in labour is the best way to feel like you're in your birthing environment. When you are now, you let the past go and let go of what could happen in the future. You take each moment of labour, one breath or one contraction at a time, while you are concentrated on the present.

WITH LOVING-KINDNESS, WORK

Oxytocin is a love hormone that is released in response to affection, love, and familiarity. Birthing with loving-kindness would almost certainly boost oxytocin and beta-endorphin levels. Between contractions, being gentle and affectionate with your partner will really help things move along and allow you to relax and let go. At births, such tenderness is common, and I have quietly stood back and allowed them to enjoy enveloping their birth and baby in love.

Remember that your baby was created out of love, and the same hormone that created your baby will also bring your baby into the world. Kissing and massaging are all beneficial. You have the right to request privacy if you feel it would help you be more intimate.

AFFIRMATIONS FOR BIRTH

Throughout your pregnancy, you would have been listening to birth affirmations. Putting those on now, along with your hypnosis songs, will help you stay in your birthing environment, whether in the background or on headphones. You can also have your partner read them to you:

- Inhale slowly and exhale slowly. I listen to and trust my body, as well as my baby.
- When I take a deep breath, I feel good. I let go as I exhaled.
- The more I relax, the softer and larger my body becomes.
- I feel more at ease the more my body softens and expands. I allow the birth energy to flow through me.
- I am focused and solid, and I draw strength from the people I love and who care for me. I am suffused with affection for my child.
- With each contraction wave, my baby, gets closer to me.
- In between contractions, my body relaxes, and during them, it stretches and opens.
- I'm in harmony with my body's rhythm, as well as the rhythm of labour.
- I picture the feeling like a soothing pressure nudging my baby down, down, down; my baby is riding the waves of labour, loving the gentle rhythm.
- As I breathe in, I relax; as I breathe out, I let go, relax.

WHEN CAN I CONTACT A MIDWIFE?

It's usually too early to call the midwife whether you're unsure if it's the right time or whether others are saying, "I guess it's time we went in." When you say, "I need to go now," it will be the right time.

People sometimes call the midwife or go to the hospital too soon after giving birth. According to studies, women frequently go to the hospital or call the midwife too fast because of their partner's or mother's fear of obligation. Although being in the hospital can make you feel better, arriving too soon increases your chances of being admitted.

When a mother is in labour, and her baby is on the way, she would be deeply absorbed in her own thoughts, not worrying about making a cup of tea for guests!

If you need reassurance, you can go to the hospital, have a scan, and either return home, or you can call the midwife, who can decide whether you should stay or go. According to studies, a pre-admission assessment for women planning a hospital birth will minimize the risk of intervention so the patient will go home feeling confident and stay at home until the time is right to return to the hospital.

WHAT IF I'M OVERDUE?

Women are put under a lot of stress because they miss their due dates, despite the fact that only about 5% of babies are delivered on their due dates. Set aside your due date and remind yourself that your baby will arrive when they are ready. Pregnancy length can vary by up to five weeks, according to research, and older mothers have longer pregnancies.

If you go past your due date, keep in mind that it's just an estimation, not the actual date your baby will be born. You would not have hit 'term' until you are 42 weeks pregnant. Just go about your business as usual, and don't feel obligated to hurry things along. Remember that allowing yourself to become anxious about it will raise your adrenaline levels, which may prevent oxytocin from rising and labour from the beginning. Did you know that you have a 95% risk of going into labour before 42 weeks and a 50% chance of going into labour between 38 and 41 weeks of pregnancy?

CHAPTER ELEVEN

MY BABY'S NEARLY HERE!

You've either contacted a midwife or arrived at the hospital. Remember, if you think you've arrived too early, you can still leave. Taking you through the basic steps of what happens when you call for a midwife or go to the hospital will help you plan and become more familiar with the procedure.

So, what happens next?

IF YOU'RE GIVING BIRTH AT HOME

On the phone, a midwife will talk with you and ask you questions about how far apart your contractions are and what's been going on. She'll almost certainly come over and take a look. She'll want to check on your baby and take some simple measurements, including your blood pressure and temperature. She may offer to perform an assessment based on your birth preferences, or she may opt to simply examine you for a while. Keep in mind that you have a say in what you agree to and don't consent to. She will wait and call another midwife if she believes you are in active labour. She might quit if she feels you have a long way to go or would benefit from some room, giving you her phone number to call if things change.

WHEN YOU GET TO THE HOSPITAL

You'll be buzzed into the labour suite when you arrive. You've probably called ahead, so they'll be expecting you. A midwife will greet you at the front desk and guide you to a room or the assessment suite. An assessment suite may be a large room with several beds, such as an award, or a small clinical side room.

The aim of the evaluation is to figure out how far along you are in your labour and how you and your baby are doing. Typically, you would be given an ultrasound at this stage to determine how much your cervix has dilated and the location of your infant. If you want to have a test, it will help to fill in the gaps in your knowledge, but it will not guarantee when your baby will be born. Always trust your intuition, even though they contradict what the midwife is telling you. If you don't want a vaginal test, you should decline it.

A clinical assessment on admission to a hospital, according to some studies, can reduce the risk of intervention. This is because if they believe you have a long way to go, they will recommend returning home. It may be comforting for some women to get that check and then go home, particularly if they live close to the hospital.

Simple tests, such as taking the temperature and blood pressure, would be made by the midwife. She can even examine you from the outside, watching how you move and breathe in response to contractions.

You will be given room to make your own when you are admitted to the facility. Make yourself at ease and ask for whatever assistance you need. Ask for what you want with confidence; part of the midwife's role is to help you in your birth wishes.

HOW DID YOU DO IT? YOUR BABY AND YOU WILL BE MONITORED

The way your labour is handled at this point is determined by many factors, including how well you and your baby are adjusting to delivery, how far along you are when admitted, and the type of midwife assigned to you.

A partogram can be filled out both in the hospital and at home to determine how the labour is going. A partogram records how much you're dilating, how long you've been in labour, the position of your cervix, the position of your fetus, your temperature, and how you're responding to labour. Anything you decide or order will also be recorded in your notes. In a hospital, you can give birth without interruption. You can still make choices that minimize interference even though your labour is high-risk and consultant-led.

AN UNINTERRUPTED BIRTH

Undisturbed birth is just what it sounds like: a birth with as little disruption as possible. Exams and checks, chatter, background noise, and lights are all examples of disturbances. By reducing these, oxytocin, the birth hormone, can circulate freely without being obstructed by adrenaline.

Trusting that the body can give birth in its own time is the foundation of mindful hypnobirthing.

Do nothing if everything is well. Keeping the number of checks and tests to a bare minimum helps your baby's birth to take place in its own time and in its own way, rather than according to charts based on averages. When you're at home, you're more likely to slip into a paradigm of uninhibited birth.

In a hospital, is it possible to give birth without being disturbed?

If you're in the hospital, you'll be able to give birth without interruption. You can always make choices to avoid interruptions and disruptions; just make sure they're on your birth preferences list. 'Just press the buzzer if you need me. Otherwise, I'll pop in every 20 minutes to do observations on you and the baby,' the midwife would usually say. If she doesn't say anything, but it sounds good to you, make sure to tell your midwife.

While the midwife may continue to chart progress on a partogram, they may begin to deviate from the guidelines, modifying their practice to assist the mother in her labour management and response. Your midwife can only interfere if she believes you or your baby are in danger. There's no reason why a hospital birth shouldn't be handled the same way a home birth would. If this is important to you, find a midwife who is willing to let things happen naturally and is interested in an uncomplicated birth.

THE MEDICALIZATION OF CHILDBIRTH

Birth is more likely to be medicalized in a hospital than at home. In a hospital setting, however, you should put measures in place to ensure that your birth is as painless as possible. Inquire with your midwife about local rules, and use what you've learned in this book to write down and express your interests. Understanding a more medical model of birth will help you make the necessary changes at any point during your baby's birth.

The progress of a woman is constantly compared to the partogram, and care decisions are made based on the image provided by the partogram rather than trusting the mother's ability to give birth to her baby in her own time and in her own way. Daily vaginal exams, typically every four hours, are needed, depending on your hospital's policies. If your labour stalls or doesn't advance as fast as your midwife or doctor would like, you might be given an amniotomy (the breaking of your waters) to speed things up.

And if you have a higher risk pregnancy and are being guided by a doctor, you should take action to ensure that your delivery is as painless as possible. Your midwife or doctor will continue to comfortably watch you and your infant, only intervening if there is a legitimate reason to do so. When all is in order, you will let the birth take its course without interfering with the speed and form of labour that your body dictates.

INTERVENTIONS

These three common interventions can affect how you feel and think during labour and delivery, as well as your physical reactions. Knowing about them and reading up on the advantages and risks will make you feel more prepared and in control of your decisions.

INDUCTION

You will be offered an induction if you go past your due dates, which is normally about 40 weeks plus ten days, but maybe sooner if you are over 35 years old. Each hospital will have its own induction policy, so it's a good idea to familiarize yourself with the one in your area. Unfortunately, induction is becoming more popular in the United Kingdom. According to an audit of 17,000 births in Aberdeen, 28% of women who were induced had no cause for induction after the birth, raising fears that women were being given intervention unnecessarily. If you force your body to go into labour before you or your baby are ready, it's possible that you're injuring yourself or your baby.

And though there is no medical cause, there may be a lot of pressure on mothers to induce labour before the due date of 42 weeks.

A pessary, which is a small tablet inserted at the cervix, is sometimes given first. Prostaglandins are released, which can stimulate labour. A balloon catheter, also known as a Foley balloon or a Cook balloon, can be used to help ripen the cervix. It's worth looking at what options are available at your local hospital and which ones could be best for you. Since sperm releases prostaglandins, sex is often recommended to kick-start labour. A drip containing artificial oxytocin may be given if a pessary or balloon catheter fails to start labour.

Artificial oxytocin does not function in the same way as your body's naturally released oxytocin, and it does not induce the release of endorphins or your body's natural analgesic. This is crucial to know if you want a birth of as little interference as possible. Labour caused by artificial oxytocin – or syntocinon as it is also called – often necessitates more focused contractions. Drip induction mothers may experience what's known as a cascade of intervention, which means that one intervention may lead to another. A drip induction, for example, may lead to pain relief options, which can lead to an epidural; epidurals, in turn, have been related to higher rates of forceps or ventouse use.

Consider how you would feel if you were told you were putting your baby at risk if you went overdue after learning about the effects of adrenaline. It can cause the stress hormones adrenaline and noradrenaline to be released, preventing the release of oxytocin and the start of labour.

The following points should be explained to women who are being offered induction of labour by healthcare professionals:

- The reasons for induction being offered.
- When, where, and how induction would take place.
- The support and pain management arrangements (recognizing that women are likely to find induced labour more painful than spontaneous labour).
- Alternatives to induction of labour if the woman prefers not to have it.
- The drawbacks and advantages of induction of labour in particular situations, as well as the induction methods suggested.
- What if the induction is unsuccessful, and what the woman's choices are in that situation.

In addition, the guidelines state:

Allowing the woman time to review the details with her husband before making a decision is important for healthcare professionals providing induction of labour.

- Encourage the woman to get facts from a variety of sources. Inviting the woman to ask questions and encouraging her to consider her choices is a good idea.
- Encourage the woman to make whatever choice she wants.

There are even more reports of women today who, after studying the facts, spoke with their healthcare provider and opted to forego induction and instead wait until their baby was ready to be born, assuming there were no medical indications for induction. This is something you can explore with your midwife.

HYPNOBIRTHING AND INDUCTION: HOW TO DO IT

Hypnobirthing strategies will assist you in being as calm as possible during your pregnancy. Accept induction for what it is until you've decided to use it, and then concentrate on creating the best possible atmosphere. To build a relaxing environment, use the anchors you've made and the MP3 tracks you've downloaded. Keep in mind that the more welcoming and relaxed you are, the easier it will be for your body to work with the induction.

MEMBRANE ARTIFICIAL RUPTURE (ARM)

If your labour is slowing down, you might be given treatments such as separating your waters (also known as an amniotomy or artificial breakup of membranes) or an amniotomy (also known as an amniotomy or artificial rupture of membranes) (ARM). This action, like anything else, has advantages and disadvantages.

Women are gradually claiming that an unwanted rupture of membranes alters the direction of their labour from one in which they were doing well to one in which they were having difficulty. An ARM also carries a variety of risks that, although minor, may significantly alter the direction of labour. 'The data indicated no shortening of the duration of the first stage of labour and a potential rise in Caesarean section,' according to a study of the available studies. Routine ARM is not recommended for labours that are progressing normally or for labours that have been prolonged'.

If your labour has slowed, think about what could have caused it.

Check your surroundings if you and the baby are fine. Is anything different now? Perhaps there has been a shift change with a new midwife; perhaps there have been some new noises; maybe you have been brought out of your 'birthing zone' for some reason. Consider oxytocin's function and how easily it can be disrupted, slowing down labour. Consider the following options for resuming labour: change your surroundings to make you feel safe and comfortable; listen to relaxing music; use hypnosis, or try aromatherapy or massage. You can also return home if all goes well. All of these things make ARM a gentle and non-invasive choice.

EXAMINATIONS OF THE VAGINAL SYSTEM

Vaginal tests may have a major influence on how the birth goes and how a mother feels. They're frequently mistaken.

You may be shocked to learn that VEs do not predict when your baby will be born, according to research. The degree to which you are dilated is not a reliable indicator of whether your baby will be born in 1 hour, 2 hours, or 5 hours. You and your baby are doing well if you and your baby are reacting well, regardless of how slowly or quickly you are dilating.

There is also something known as a plateau, where you may continue to have contractions without dilating for up to five hours, according to science. Keep cool if anything happens to you! Go for it if you're feeling good and the baby is doing well. Things are always progressing; it's not only about the cervix opening; it's also about how it softens and thins. Each contraction assists the baby is moving into the best position for birth.

Here are some ideas for making vaginal exams more pleasant:

- Get any tests done by the same midwife. According to research, measurements taken on the same woman by different people can vary significantly; in some cases, the discrepancy can be as much as 2 cm.
- If you're having an intervention, make sure to breathe deeply and relax. Put your headphones on, and don't feel compelled to engage in small talk or conversation.
- Request only the most basic tests. Studies suggest that doing an exam at a unit before being admitted reduces the risk of intervention, but there may be no need for further tests unless there is a medical indication.
- You have the choice of not knowing how dilated you are. Finding out you're 4 cm can be demoralizing for some women, and it's at this stage that they seek pain relief. In reality, if you're 4 cm, you might be 7 cm in a matter of hours. Women dilate in a variety of ways.
- Have faith in your body's ability to labour at a safe and appropriate rate for you.
- Did you know that the appearance of a red/purple line running from your anus and extending between your buttocks can be used to measure cervical dilation? According to research, a significant percentage of women experience this. Without an internal examination, this will provide a clear indicator of dilation and how far down your baby's head is. As an option, you should speak with your midwife about it.
- If you're offered a vaginal examination, some good questions to ask are: Is there a medical reason for me to have one right now?
- What impact will this have on my treatment?

- Why do I need to know my current dilated pupil size? Is it possible to postpone it? Is there any other way for me to learn more?

CAN HYPNOSIS BE EFFECTIVE?

To be honest, what do you think? Yes, it certainly would. Hypnosis is a highly effective type of anesthesia that is used in surgery all over the world. This excerpt depicts Dr. John Butler hypnotizing himself for a hernia operation. It can make you uncomfortable to read, but it demonstrates what your mind is capable of.

WHAT IF I NEED ADDITIONAL PAIN RELIEF?

If you're going to get a hypnobirthing, you could have moved away from the pain-relieving paradigm. Someone once told me that if a woman can sit still long enough for an epidural during labour, she can definitely give birth without them; all she needs is the right help.

After weighing the costs and benefits, there can be occasions when taking pharmacological pain relief is the best option for you. If you are adamant about not having a forceps birth, for example, you should think about the effects of an epidural, which can increase the chances of having an assisted birth by 50%.

If you need any pain treatment choices for some purpose, you can make them with a clear understanding of why you're doing so. Knowing the effects of such interventions also ensures you understand how they can affect a normal birth. Natural and pharmacological pain management strategies are listed below. Non-pharmacological procedures, by definition, carry fewer risks since they are non-invasive.

PAIN RELIEF BY NATURAL MEANS

TENS

TENS is a system that uses a series of tiny pads with electrodes that you attach to your lower back skin. It stimulates the nerve endings in that region by sending tiny electrical impulses into them. If you visualize the neural pathways as one-lane roads that can only accommodate one car at a time, electrical impulses occupy certain roads, essentially blocking the road and preventing the sensation of a contraction from passing. They can be purchased or rented in some stores.

The gateway pain theory underpins TENS. Although it is unclear how it works, it has been shown to have a powerful placebo effect (meaning that if you believe it is turned on when it isn't, you will experience the same or similar effects as if it were). I know a few women who swear by it as a source of stability and attention. It aids some women in diverting their attention away from their contractions. If you're going to use TENS, make sure you practice with your partner first because they can be fiddly. Make sure your partner knows how to use it when it's turned on. If you inquire, you may be able to persuade your partner to turn it up. If you want to have a water birth, keep in mind that you won't be able to bring the TENS pump into the pool with you.

AROMATHERAPY

At some points during labour, aromatherapy oils can be very helpful. Oils like clary sage, lavender, and mandarin are often used to help women relax or speed up labour. Pressure is reduced as the muscles relax. During your pregnancy, you should see an aromatherapist who can help you develop an oil that is tailored to your own emotions and birth expectations.

An aromatherapist can also have specific guidance on what is and is not safe to use. Aromatherapy is used by midwives in some hospitals; ask your midwife if this is available in your area.

MUSCLE MASSAGE

Massage can make you feel more connected and supported during labour by reducing discomfort and increasing your sense of connection. During labour, your partner will learn how to massage your knees, lower back, and shoulders.

REFLEXOLOGY AND ACUPRESSURE

Simple acupressure and reflexology points can be learned. Make an appointment with a pregnancy reflexologist or an acupuncturist if this is something that concerns you. They will help you learn about essential acupressure points to use during labour. Alternatively, there are a plethora of online tools that will show you how to identify pressure points on the body that are useful during contractions.

WATER

Water is a common natural pain reliever during labour that works well with mindful hypnobirthing. A pool or a bath can be relaxing, but a shower can also be soothing. You should sit in the tub with a chair and let the water cascade over your stomach. Swimming can be beneficial to some women, but it may also delay labour in others. If this happens to you, simply get out of the house, warm up, and relax. Remember to remain calm if it does slow down.

Simply complete your workouts, relax, and sleep if you are able. When you're ready, your contractions will begin again. If you are at home and before going to the hospital, you can also take a bath. Ask your partner to pour water over your bump or back, whether you're in a pool or a bath; this can be very calming and relaxing. If you're planning a home birth or just want to relax before going to the hospital, you can buy or rent a pool to have in your own home; you may not want to get out and drive!

HOMEOPATHY

For certain women, using homeopathy to manage feelings and sensations during labour may be beneficial. Many homeopaths have a pregnancy and labour consultation, which includes the loaning of a homeopathic birth kit.

DOULA

A doula has a plethora of tools and tricks up her sleeve to assist with labour and delivery. According to research, having a doula or continuous support during labour decreases the need for pharmacological pain relief.

GAS AND AIR

The mixture of nitrous oxide and oxygen in gas and air is 50% nitrous oxide and 50% oxygen. It's inhaled through a small inhaler, has a quick impact, and disperses in less than 60 seconds. This is why, as soon as a contraction begins to rise, women are told to take a breath and then stop as the contraction subsides. Entonox is another name for it. There is very little evidence that gas and air have a harmful effect on your infant. Using the deepener or 3, 2, 1, relax, relax, relax, between contractions.

MEPTID (OPIOIDS), DIAMORPHINE, AND PETHIDINE

You've been advised to avoid alcohol and some foods for nine months, but you're given morphine during labour! These medications cross the placenta and may have an effect on your infant, though Meptid is thought to have fewer side effects. If your baby is born too soon after this medication is given, it may cause respiratory problems and require special care.

When a mother has taken an opioid, her baby can become drowsy, which can affect breastfeeding. Both of these medications can cause vomiting in one out of every three women and make you feel disoriented. Some women complain they feel out of control and are unable to speak or articulate their desires easily, whereas others say it has been beneficial to them.

EPIDURAL

A local anesthetic injected into the cerebrospinal fluid is known as an epidural. It's a powerful pain reliever, but it can have a big impact on the amount of labour you have. You can be confined to your bed if you have an epidural. A very low dose can allow you to move around the bed if you're lucky, but getting out of bed would be difficult.

It may cause the second stage of labour to take longer because your muscles aren't working as hard to shift your baby into the proper place to descend. When combined with lying down, this may reduce the pelvic outlet by up to 30%, which is why epidurals lead to more ventouse or forceps births. Other side effects include losing bladder control and possibly requiring a catheter.

An epidural headache, which is a serious headache, affects one out of every 100 women. You have not 'failed' hypnobirthing if you opt for an epidural.

Remember that the aim of hypnobirthing is for you to have the best possible birth experience. You are hypnobirthing if you have weighed the risks and made the decision that you believe is best for you. If you have an epidural, a helpful tip for your husband is to make sure you have low lighting, massages and feel loved and cared for as much as possible. Many people I've met who have had an epidural have said that this part of the birth vanished after the epidural and that it altered their experience. Keep it special!

Final Stages of Labour

If you're in the hospital, you've probably arrived just in time for your baby to be born. You'll be deep in your birthing zone in the final stages of labour, allowing the contractions to pass through you while concentrating on your breathing. Your partner should have already begun preparing the room at the hospital or at home in the manner that you had arranged with your anchors from previous chapters.

If you've just arrived at the hospital and things are moving fast, you won't have much time to make improvements to your bed. Your contractions may get closer together as you get closer to giving birth to your baby; they may even feel like they're coming in waves on top of each other. You can also hit a point where your body needs to rest for up to 30 minutes before moving your baby down the vaginal canal. This stage is also known as the "rest and be grateful" stage.

Your body's hormones spontaneously change at this point in labour to raise adrenaline levels while decreasing oxytocin levels. In the early stages of labour, adrenaline levels should be very low; but, when your cervix is almost completely dilated, normally about 7–10 cm, you can experience a normal surge of adrenaline. The term "transition" is used to describe this point. This primitive reaction makes a woman more alert, and if you were an animal in the wild, it would be a sign that you should find a safe place to give birth because your baby is on its way. This final burst of adrenaline also benefits your baby: their white blood count rises, improving their immunity; blood flow to the brain, heart, and kidneys rises, preparing them to function; and it helps your baby's lungs prepare for that first breath.

WHAT IF LABOUR SLOWS DOWN?

If your labour slows down, consider your surroundings first. Is anything different now? Is your anxiety getting the best of you? Do you have a new midwife on your team? Is it getting louder? Disturbances or changes will raise your alertness, lowering oxytocin levels and slowing your contractions.

If this occurs, remain cool. There's no need to rush anything if you and your baby are in good health. Make the most of the time by lying on your left side in bed, relaxed with your pillow and blanket and your companion nearby. Put on your hypnosis tracks and float away. You may also use the special position visualization that you and your partner have practiced.

BREATHE YOUR CHILD INTO THE WORLD.

You may have read or seen stories of women turning red in the face as a result of pushing. That doesn't have to be the case. The Valsalva Manoeuvre is the sustained chin on the chest, deep breath, hold, and push school of thought, and it is now considered to increase the risk of complications in the second level. For both you and your son, it will lower oxygen levels and raise carbon dioxide levels. According to studies, the duration of the second stage is unaffected.

You won't need to be told to push; your body will tell you when it's time. Follow the body's instructions. Maintain your concentration in your birthing zone.

And if you know you're 10 cm dilated, just keep breathing and breathing and breathing, following your body's rhythm. It's possible that you'll notice your baby going down before the midwife does. Your body will help to carry your baby to you in a normal peristaltic movement while you breathe and relax, breathe and relax. Peristalsis is the movement that your intestines and bowel muscles make as they pass food across your body. It's like a gentle pulsing wave nudges your baby down and down. If you feel compelled to drive, do so, but remember to take deep breaths in between.

MEETING YOUR BABY

One of the most incredible moments of your life could be the moment your baby slips into the world and onto your chest. You've completed the mission! You have cherished, nurtured, and grown the little bundle of baby you are holding in your arms for the past nine months. You are more than likely attached to your baby in ways you are unaware of. As your baby enters the world, adrenaline levels drop, and oxytocin levels increase, ensuring that you and your baby are surrounded by beta-endorphins and happiness–this aids in the formation of a bond between you and your child. If you intend to breastfeed, your baby can latch on within a few minutes of birth, or it may take longer. Whatever happens, take it all in stride, remain calm, and enjoy looking at and tuning in to your kid.

Don't worry about measuring your baby; it won't change in the next hour, and the midwife will be able to measure your baby when they're snuggled up against you.

This 'Golden Hour' is a priceless opportunity to bond and communicate with your baby through your body and mind.

Take a picture, but keep your distance from Facebook and Twitter! These are priceless moments after birth. You will never be able to bring them back. The feel of your baby's soft skin, meeting their eyes, and holding them tucked up in your arms are all things that should be remembered. You won't be able to remember the memory if you aren't completely immersed in it.

When your baby takes in the world outside the womb for the first time, you, your baby, and your partner are sharing a special and personal moment. Make sure you have a picture, but several midwives have recently stated that they want to prohibit phones from being used during births. Mothers are texting, sending Twitter alerts, posting on their Facebook walls, and sending pictures to friends before the placenta has arrived, missing out on those vital bonding moments. Before they leave the hospital, several babies now have a digital imprint.

I know you'll want to tell everyone but set aside an hour for yourself, your partner, and your baby to reconnect and bond. In that hour, get to know your kid.

THE FINAL STAGE

The third stage of childbirth is when the placenta is delivered. You will experience what is known as a 'physiological third stage' in an uncomplicated birth. This means that instead of making a placenta injection to hasten its delivery, you let the body release it naturally. Breastfeeding and skin-to-skin contact may help to release the placenta by causing the uterus to contract and release oxytocin. The cord ceases pulsing, begins to lengthen, and the uterus contracts and releases the placenta due to the gradual release of oxytocin and prolactin.

The natural birth of the placenta will take anywhere from minutes to over an hour for certain women. The majority of them take between 10 and 20 minutes. Some women choose to consume their placenta after birth as a smoothie or in specially prepared capsules, a process known as "placenta encapsulation." This is because studies have shown that hormonal concentrations in the placenta can help with milk supply, minimize post-partum depression, and increase energy levels. It has pain-relieving properties, according to early experiments in rats.

In certain cultures, such as Malaysia, the placenta is buried, giving the genetically similar tissue to the baby the proper burial it deserves.

You will be given an injection to help the uterus contract and release the placenta in a medicalized third stage. Delayed cord clamping, also known as "waiting for white," helps the baby to obtain more blood from the placenta, which has been shown to be beneficial to the baby's health. Even if you have a managed third stage or if your baby is born early or, in some cases, by Caesarean, you can still ask for the cord to be left until it stops pulsing. If you have any complications during pregnancy or childbirth, a controlled third stage might be prescribed.

CHAPTER TWELVE

WHEN THINGS TAKE A DIFFERENT PATH

I'll go through some of the unexpected choices and complications that women can face during labour in this chapter. These will give you an idea of how conscientious hypnobirthing strategies can be used in a variety of situations, as well as how couples make decisions and manage their birth journey. Every woman is unique, and birth will throw you a curveball, forcing you to reconsider your priorities and presenting you with options at a fork in the road. This could be anything from the baby's location to a Caesarean birth.

You won't really know the circumstances and reasons why you made a choice if you have to make an unusual choice due to the path your birth has taken. Our memories are unreliable, particularly when we make decisions based on emotion and possibly fear, and hindsight can paint a very different image.

Take a deep breath and think about the exercise and your BRAINS questions. If anything happens when you're pregnant, you'll have plenty of time to look into it. And if you're in the early stages of childbirth, your partner can do some online research to support you with your questions.

However, and during labour and delivery, you will have plenty of opportunities to ask questions and possibly do your own analysis.

If you make a decision that you think you'll come to regret later, make sure you have time to think about these three things.

If you have the opportunity, write them down. It will serve as a reminder that you did your best with the knowledge you had at the time:

These are the facts that were presented to me.

This is the decision I came to.

These are the factors that influenced my decision.

Many of the options that occur have alternatives, as shown by the following examples of common complications. They also demonstrate how the hypnosis methods you learned in this book can serve you well in any situation.

PLACENTA IN A LOW-LYING POSITION

Many women believe that practicing hypnobirthing is pointless if they are advised at their 20-week ultrasound that their placenta is low-lying and that they may need a Caesarean birth. If your placenta does not cover the womb's neck, however, there is unlikely to be a problem. Consider your uterus to be a deflated balloon, and place a small piece of Blu Tack close, but not over, the balloon's neck. Now go ahead and blow it up. You'll notice that as the balloon grows larger, the Blu Tack piece travels farther away from the balloon's neck. The same can be said for how your uterus develops. In the word, a condition known as placenta praevia is extremely rare. Around 98 percent of women who have a low-lying placenta at their 20-week ultrasound will have a perfectly normal pregnancy at term.

And if you have to have a Caesarean birth, the hypnosis methods you practice would help you and your infant, so it's well worth practicing them if you've been told you have a low-lying placenta.

BREECH AND POSTERIOR POSITION OF THE BABY

The cervix will dilate more rapidly, and the baby will move down if the baby is in a good place for delivery. Often babies are in more unusual positions, such as breech (head up) or back to back (baby's back facing backward instead of forwards). You can help prevent this by sitting properly during pregnancy; stop slouching on a sofa and instead find places where your back is straight, and you are slightly leaning forward. Sitting at a desk with a birth ball can be really relaxing. Depending on the condition of the breach, you might be able to have a vaginal birth if your baby is breech. Breech births are becoming more common in hospitals.

Remember that if your baby is breech, they can switch at any time. Relax, listen to your hypnosis songs, and trust that your baby will do what is best for him or her.

Active movement during labour may help the baby get into a good position, particularly if the baby's back is aligned with yours. Movement, such as rocking or bouncing on a birthing ball, is a safer choice than lying down on a bed because it makes it harder for the baby to swizzle into the right place for birth.

A visit to a chiropractor or an osteopath who specializes in birth can be extremely beneficial prior to labour, simply to correct any misalignments.

MEMBRANE RUPTURE THAT HAPPENS TOO SOON (PROM)

Waters split before labour begins in around 8–12% of full-term pregnancies starting at 37 weeks. Premature rupture of membranes is the medical term for this (PROM). Within 24 hours, about 95% of women would go into labour on their own. To minimize the risk of infection, most hospitals have a procedure of inducing someone after 24 hours. Remember that this is a strategy, not a requirement. You must balance the true risk of infection against the risks of induction, particularly if you want to have an uncomplicated birth. According to research, the disparity in neo-natal infection between induction and expectant management rises by 0.5 to 1%. Waiting but making simple observations is the task of expectant management.

If you refuse to be induced, you will be told of the infection risk.

- Be informed that you should give birth in a hospital.
- It is recommended that you remain in for 12 hours after the birth for observation.

EXPECTANT MANAGEMENT

If you want to wait, your midwife or the hospital can advise you to • Check your temperature every four hours and notify your midwife or the hospital if your temperature is above 37.4 degrees Celsius, if you are feeling unwell, or if the color or scent of your waters changes. Every 24 hours, have a midwife check the fetal heart rate and activity.

- If you are not in labour after 72 hours, see an obstetrician for a consultation.

If you order it, your midwife will arrange for an induction.

BLOOD PRESSURE IS HIGH

Throughout your pregnancy, your blood pressure will be monitored on a regular basis. Increased blood pressure has been linked to complications, including pre-eclampsia, which is why it should be tested on a regular basis. And if the blood pressure rises above 140/60 or is followed by other signs, would a midwife be worried.

White Coat Syndrome is the most serious issue that women face. This is when the heart starts pounding as a result of fear while having tests performed at a doctor's office. According to research, women are more likely to develop White Coat Syndrome during pregnancy, with up to 32% of pregnant women being affected. When your blood pressure is taken, use your hypnosis methods to relax and calm yourself if you have elevated blood pressure without any other signs. If your blood pressure rises at term, your doctor can recommend an induction.

GOING OVER YOUR DATES

One of the most common reasons for an intervention in the form of induction is going over your dates. Babies arrive at their own pace; if all goes well, your baby will need a little more time. When both of you are ready, your body will initiate labour. Do a lot of study before committing to induction and really consider the consequences of induction against waiting.

If you want a natural birth, you should think about how an induction would affect your treatment and the birth. With induction, you can have a regular vaginal birth without drugs, but it can be more difficult than going into labour naturally, and the chance of a cascade of interventions is higher.

It is also more traumatic because some women become very nervous about the procedure, causing their bodies to fight back by entering the fear-tension-pain loop. If you're being inducted for some cause, the only thing you can do is lean in; once you've made your decision, embrace it and use your techniques. The key is to take breaks when you can and concentrate on remaining in your birthing zone. You can also dim the lights, play music, use a birthing ball, and use as many hypnobirthing methods as you want.

PRE-TERM LABOUR

It's considered pre-term labour if you go into labour before 37 weeks. You may not be induced if your waters split before 37 weeks, but the doctor will use expectant management, and you will be expected to remain in the hospital. You will be closely watched and may be given steroid injections to help your baby's lungs develop. If this occurs, the hypnosis methods you have mastered may be extremely beneficial. They will not only help you relax, but they will also support your kid. Use what you've learned in this book to prepare for premature birth. There has been a lot of research done on this, and it shows that the baby can still get oxygen through the cord – this is particularly vital for a premature baby.

Speak to your care team about having as much skin-on-skin time as possible if your baby is born and goes to the Special Care Baby Unit (SCBU) or Neo-Natal Unit. This has been shown to be beneficial to both you and your son. In reality, some hospitals are opting for this over incubators. You can use the hypnosis tracks to get some rest and relaxation while waiting for your baby to be brought to you on the ward.

CHAPTER THIRTEEN

WELCOME HOME

Depending on your birth and the hospital, you can leave anywhere from hours to days after your baby is born if you had a hospital birth. You have the option of being discharged within hours if your labour was fast and painless. You would need to remain in longer if you had a Caesarean birth or an intervention.

When you are at home, the midwife will leave after everything has been cleared up and she is satisfied that both of your and your baby's tests have been completed successfully. Then you can cuddle up in bed with your baby and enjoy him or her.

THE FOURTH TRIMESTER

The 'fourth trimester' refers to the days and weeks after your baby's birth. This is a time to take it easy, embrace life at a slower pace, and adjust to life as a newly expanded family. Being prepared for this process before the birth of your child will put you in a great position and make it much easier to transition from birth to the early days without feeling like you're still catching up.

Even if they were well prepared for the pregnancy, new parents are frequently unprepared for the fourth trimester. This step can be made much simpler by slowing down and limiting what you do. You can use this period of calm to engage mindfully with your baby and get to know them without being distracted.

Your baby will be soothed if you remain cool. Your baby will imitate you and be constantly conscious of you. The strategies you learned for the birth will also support you in the days and weeks following the birth. Your breathing exercises and the '3, 2, 1 relax, relax, relax' exercise will help you center yourself.

GETTING A GLIMPSE OF REALITY DURING THE EARLY WEEKS

Remember, at the end of the day, all your baby wants is your love, your cuddles, and your warmth. You'll discover that parenting entails surrender and, at times, compromises in order to care for this vulnerable child; this may feel like it's done at your own cost, both physically and emotionally. It is, however, an amazing, stunning, and unique experience. Your baby will steal your breath away at unpredictable times, and those are priceless moments.

It's like embarking on a journey that requires you to brace yourself in order to make room for you as a parent and your child to develop. You wouldn't take a long trip in your car unless it was serviced, washed, and loaded with the absolute necessities. You'd have a schedule and know where to stop along the way. Surely you'd like to take a break and take in the sights along the way? If the car had a flat tire or needed to be repaired, you'd have someone to contact.

WOULDN'T YOU BE READY FOR ANYTHING?

Preparing for the days, weeks, and months following your baby's birth will be extremely helpful to you as you mature into the mother you will become. Finding the room inside and around you to sink into the final moments of pregnancy will help you begin to make changes and, most importantly, feel at ease with slowing down. Slowing down rather than jumping on the brakes allows for a far smoother transition in a world where 'busy-ness' is valued.

Having a baby is a life-changing event; not only does your body change, but your brain changes as well, preparing you for life as a mother. Things can feel like a rollercoaster emotionally and physically, and being prepared can make things a lot simpler. A healthy postnatal plan and support system will also help to lower the risk of postnatal depression and anxiety.

PREPARING FOR LIFE AFTER BIRTH

We are becoming more conscious of the importance of caring for a mother postnatal as a result of research – studies show how a lack of care, exhaustion, and anxiety can have a significant effect on new mothers' health, disrupting the early bonding experience. It's important to keep in mind that postnatal plans are essential.

COMING UP WITH A POSTNATAL PLAN

Consider what would make life easier for you after the baby is born. The truth is that both you and your partner will be exhausted. You can need some time to recover, relax, and reconnect with your baby and partner. You can need assistance, and a small group of loving, trustworthy friends and family can be extremely beneficial. It's great if you want to go out as soon as possible but plan ahead, so you don't have to if you don't feel like it.

Self-care is always the first thing to go after you have a newborn, and having a postnatal plan will help you prepare to look after your mental and physical well-being. It will provide a safety net if you find it difficult to concentrate on your immediate needs after giving birth. Consider the following: practical planning, encouragement, and self-care.

PRACTICAL PREPARATION

- I'm sure you have all of your baby's clothing, a cot, and a stroller, but what about the rest?
- Make a few freezer-friendly recipes.

- Schedule an online grocery order for at least the first eight weeks. Consider how you'll maintain a schedule for the other kids. Who can help, and how can they help?
- If possible, make sure all bills, renewals, and insurances are current, and schedule an answering machine message or a door sign. Consider how you can share household responsibilities and who can assist you.
- People are always eager to help, so start thinking about who you should ask and what you'll need now.
- Inquire with friends about what they may be able to assist with, especially when they come to visit.
- Accept help gladly if it is provided, such as making lunch, doing the laundry, or getting groceries.
- Create visiting hours to secure your sleeping time.
- Make a list of phone numbers for people you may call for advice or help.

If you plan to breastfeed, keep the phone numbers of a nearby breastfeeding counsellor or a telephone service like La Leche handy. The sooner you seek help, the better.

SELF-CARE

The importance of self-care cannot be overstated. And if it seems like there isn't enough time, you should prepare ahead.

CONCLUSION

We have come to the end of this book; kindly note that if everything said in this book is taking into consideration, then you are ready for free and painless birth. Let's take a short preview about what hypnobirthing does;

1. The baby's ideal place

Your baby should be in a good place for easier labour: head-down and facing forwards, not with its back to your back and using your front as a hammock. Daily yoga exercises on all fours are part of hypnobirthing to support this perfect "anterior position," which helps you not to slump on the couch for hours. Sit up straight (at work and at home) and take a stroll as much as you can.

2. Have faith in your birth partner

Every expectant mother deserves her birth partner's undivided attention and unwavering support. Do hypnobirthing with them and write your birth plan with them so that they can intervene and make decisions on your behalf if necessary.

3. Get rid of your worries

Maggie Howell recommends writing down any concerns you have or negative feedback you encounter in the weeks leading up to your baby's birth in order to feel more comfortable and calm. Actively let them go by imagining tying them to a helium balloon and watching them float free or writing them down and burning the paper to let them go symbolically.

4. Be careful not to tear.

It's normal to need an episiotomy (a cut made by a doctor or midwife) or have a tear down there during childbirth, but there are ways to minimize the chances. Hypnobirthing teaches you how to prepare for your birth by doing pelvic floor exercises and perineal massage on a daily basis. To stop straining during the transition stage of labour, instead of being ordered to "press" by the midwife, try to loosen and relax your muscles while panting with your breath. This, combined with your previous perineum massage and pelvic floor exercises, should help your skin stretch rather than tear.

5. Make a movement during labour

Hip circles, 'rocking and rolling,' and 'grape treading' not only reinforce the optimal position for the baby in labour, but the movement also helps the circulation and hormones circulate, and it can release lactic acid buildup, preventing stress (which makes contractions more painful).

6. Use the 'wave theory to solve the problem.

You will feel more at ease at home in a familiar setting during the first stage of labour, but if you feel the need to go to the hospital and your contractions are thick and fast, follow the 'wave theory': dive in and don't fight it. Relax the muscles; if you tense up in some way, the contractions will be more intense, and the labour will take longer.

7. Build a pleasant working atmosphere

You just need to look at how other mammals give birth to understanding why privacy is ideal, as Katherine Graves points out. They retreat to a tiny, secure space where only they are at ease. Hypnobirthing is based on the idea that we should also indulge our desires for intimacy. Low lighting, a warm temperature, music if you like it or silence if you don't, and calming scents like lavender oil on tissue are all things to ask for. You can discover a variety of massage methods that your birthing partner can use to relax and distract you.

8. Your breath is crucial.

The deep breathing that is slow, steady, and rhythmic will assist you in your labour. We advised inhaling for energy and courage as well as oxygen and exhaling for release - the secret to getting your baby out! Sighing and yawning often produce endorphins, which are natural pain relievers. Make low, deep noises when you breathe instead of the high-pitched, breathy sounds you hear in movies, which would only help to frighten yourself. We shared visualization strategies for 'up breathing' (to use during contractions, or surges as she refers to them in the first stage of labour) and 'down breathing' (to use during the second stage of labour) (for the second stage, when the baby is entering the world). The vaginal tissue will get smoother and suppler as you breathe deeper, making it easier for the baby to move down the birth canal.

9. Stop lying down as much as possible.

Avoid lying down for doctor's tests (to see how dilated the baby's head is, for example), as this will slow down the labour. The optimal position for labour is to be upright, dealing with gravity, so suggest lying on your side. Lying down like a stranded beetle prevents the sacrum and coccyx from tipping back and opening, which can lengthen your labour. That's not ideal!

10. Effectively manage pain

Hypnobirthing encourages you to reconsider the word "pain" and think of labour as "effective pain" (pain that serves a purpose) and a catalyst for the mothering process. "Sensations of pressure, strength, and warmth," Maggie Howell explains contractions. To cope, she recommends relaxing your jaw and shoulders, breathing deeply, and counting to yourself "3, 2, 1 relax." Aside from natural pain relievers like gas and air, a water tub, and a T.E.N.S system, consider visualizations to help you control your emotions. Imagine going to a special place in your mind, such as a tropical beach, and reliving a vacation or special experience, or imagine tuning into your inner remote control and turning down the feeling of pain to a manageable number and feeling. Accept the intense sensations as a warning that you are about to meet your baby in the final stages of labour. Know that the endorphins will (hopefully!) help you forget about any pain you might have experienced. Mother Nature knows what she's doing.

Congratulations once again on reading this book. PEACE!!!

CPSIA information can be obtained
at www.ICGtesting.com
Printed in the USA
BVHW051446050123
655630BV00012B/855